Service-Based Learning

acute general medicine

SELF-ASSESSMENT WORKBOOK

Edited by Kumar and Clark

Open University Centre for Education in Medicine
Royal College of Physicians
Hospital Doctor

acute general medicine **SELF-ASSESSMENT WORKBOOK**

is available from:

Reed Healthcare Publishing
Quadrant House
The Quadrant
Sutton
Surrey SM2 5AS

Telephone 020 8652 8789
Email: Hospital.doctor@rbi.co.uk

ISBN 1 873207 07 7

Published by:
Reed Business Information
Quadrant House
The Quadrant
Sutton
Surrey SM2 5AS

Laid out and typeset by: Brian Cronk Design
Printed by: Interprint Limited Malta

How to use the workbook

Service-Based Learning for Acute General Medicine is based on the Royal College of Physicians' Core Curriculum for Senior House Officers in General (Internal) Medicine, looking specifically at the cases that would be encountered on-take.

Service-Based Learning is a way of organising your training so that:

- You get the most educational benefit from the post
- You review your practical experience systematically
- There are practice-related learning materials available to you
- You have the opportunity for self-assessment of your learning

Service-Based Learning consists of four types of learning which are based on your service experience and relate to the curriculum.

Using Service-Based Learning

To get the most from Service-Based Learning you will need to use both the Brief Learning Materials and the Self-assessment Workbook. This workbook provides a checklist linked to the topics for Acute General Medicine for you to keep a record of your four types of Service-Based Learning which are explained below:

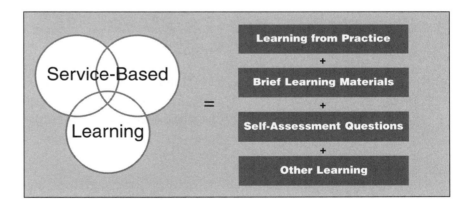

Learning from Practice

We are aware that doctors in training learn most from the patients they see when they see them, in preparation and with follow-up.

You can use the list of topics at the front of the workbook to keep a record that you have seen a particular acute case.

Brief Learning Materials (BLMs)

These materials are organised into groups to cover all acute general medicine topics. Each short piece should take around 10-15 minutes to digest and is designed to help in the immediate understanding and management of a patient. With this in mind their presentation is practice based with examples. They can also be used in preparation and follow-up as well as for learning about a new topic.

You can use the list of topics at the front of the workbook to keep a record of the BLMs you have used.

Self-Assessment Questions (SAQs)

The Self-Assessment Questions and Model Answers relate directly to each group of BLMs and are contained in this workbook. You can use them to check your understanding of the topics covered by the BLMs in a number of ways. They are valuably used in weekly educational meetings where the answers are discussed amongst all members of the team. They are also frequently used for home study and on their own to test gaps in learning.

You can use the list of topics at the front of the workbook to keep a record of the SAQs you have completed.

Other Learning

You will also find a column in the list of topics for other learning, You can put a mark here if you'd like to record other types of learning such as observations, educational meetings and events or personal study time.

List of Authors

Dr Simon Alywin	Prof Parveen Kumar
Dr Roger Amos	Dr John McAuley
Dr Janet Anderson	Dr Adam McLean
Dr Veronique Bataille	Dr Karim Meeran
Dr Mark Caulfield	Dr Heather Milburn
Dr Michael Clark	Dr David Paige
Dr Charles Clarke	Dr K John Pasi
Dr Craig Davidson	Dr Stephen Patchett
Dr Christopher Davidson	Dr Drew Provan
Dr Keren Davies	Dr M R Qadiri
Dr David DíCruz	Dr G S Raj
Dr Noemi Eiser	Dr Mark Rake
Dr Ian Fawcett	Dr Armine Sefton
Dr Tim Gluck	Dr David Trash
Dr Martin Hurst	Dr David Watson
Dr Gordon Jackson	Dr Mark Weaver
Dr Ramesh C Joshi	Dr Peter White
Dr Mark Kinirons	Dr Peter Wilkinson

Other contributors

Dr James Ahlquist	Dr Des Johnston
Dr John Amess	Dr Peter Kopelman
Dr David Blainey	Dr David Leaver
Dr Bob Bown	Dr Brian Livesley
Dr T Briggs	Dr Fiona Moss
Dr Mac Cochrane	Dr Christina Williams
Dr Mark Cottee	Dr Jennifer Worrall
Dr Lucy Goundry	

Acknowledgements

Serviced Based Learning in acute general medicine could not have been developed without the hard work of all involved in defining the topics of the Brief Learning Materials (BLMs), writing the BLMs, short answer questions and answers and in piloting the scheme. All are Members and Fellows of the Royal College of Physicians.

We would like to thank the postgraduate department of Barts and the London NHS Trust and the Director of North Thames, Dr Elisabeth Paice, for the initial financing of the project. Hospital Doctor took over the funding and the production of the final materials. The Open University Centre for Education in Medicine, who started the concept of SBL, co-ordinated the project on a daily basis. We would like to particularly thank Claire Waring, Julian Mack and Clare Jennings for their enormous hard work, help and continued enthusiasm. The Royal College of Physicians helped to establish the project by hosting the initial meeting and reviewing each of its stages.

Project team

Project director	Prof Janet Grant
Editors	Prof Parveen Kumar, Dr Michael Clark
Project manager	Claire Waring
Production co-ordinator	Phil Johnson

Contents

Q   A

List of topics for Serviced-Based Learning in Acute General Medicine

You can use this list to keep a record of your four different types of Service-Based Learning	Learnt from practice	BLM used	SAQ completed	Other learning undertaken
Group 1 Infectious diseases				
Item 1: Pyrexia of unknown origin (PUO)				
Item 2: Septicaemia				
Item 3: Meningococcal meningitis and septicaemia				
Item 4: Pseudomembranous colitis				
Item 5: Food poisoning – E. Coli 0157				
Item 6: Typhoid				
Item 7: Returning traveller				
Item 8: Shingles				
Item 9: Epstein-Barr virus				
Group 2 STDs				
Item 1: HIV/Aids				
Group 3 Nutrition				
Item 1: Feeding the patient				
Group 4 Gastroenterology				
Item 1: Vomiting				
Item 2: Weight loss				
Item 3: Hiccups				
Item 4: Dysphagia				
Item 5: Constipation				
Item 6: Diarrhoea				
Item 7: Abdominal pain				
Item 8: Dyspepsia				
Item 9: Peptic ulcer disease				
Item 10: Iron deficiency anaemia				
Item 11: Rectal bleeding				
Item 12: Family history of colon cancer				
Item 13: Functional bowel disease				
Group 5 Liver, biliary and pancreatic disorders				
Item 1: Abnormal liver function tests				
Item 2: Jaundice				
Item 3: Acute liver disease				
Item 4: Ascites				
Item 5: Haematemesis and melaena				
Item 6: Liver failure				
Item 7: Alcohol abuse				
Item 8: Cholecystitis				

	Learnt from practice	BLM used	SAQ completed	Other learning undertaken
Group 6 **Haematology and Oncology**				
Item 1: Microcytic and macrocytic anaemia				
Item 2: Haemolytic anaemia				
Item 3: Sickle cell crisis				
Item 4: Elevated haemoglobin (polycythaemia)				
Item 5: Elevated white blood cell count				
Item 6: Elevated platelet count				
Item 7: Glucose-6-phosphate dehydrogenase deficiency				
Item 8: Bleeding disorders				
Item 9: Platelet disorders				
Item 10: Thrombosis				
Item 11: Splenomegaly, splenectomy and hyposplenism				
Item 12: Blood transfusion				
Item 13: Haematological Oncology				
Item 14: Anaemia in rheumatoid arthiritis				
Item 15: Anaemia in chronic renal failure				
Item 16: Anaemia in liver disease				
Item 17: Cancer				
Item 18: Infection/sepsis				
Group 7 **Geriatrics**				
Item 1: Blackout				
Item 2: Falls in the elderly				
Item 3: Delirium				
Item 4: Dementia				
Item 5: Depression				
Item 6: Non-specific presentation of illness in the elderly				
Item 7: Appropriate assessment scales				
Item 8: Stroke				
Item 9: Heart disease in the elderly				
Item 10 Transient ischaemic attack				
Item 11: Hypothermia				
Item 12: Pressure sores				
Item 13: Urinary tract infection and incontinence				
Item 14: Elements of provisional discharge plan				
Item 15: Options for elderly patients who cannot return home				
Item 16: Acute hot joint				
Item 17: Parkinson's Disease				
Item 18: Drug treatment in older people/drug treatment as a cause of illness and admission to hospital				
Item 19: Do not resuscitate (DNR) decision-making				
Group 8 **Rheumatology**				
Item 1: Osteoarthritis (OA)				
Item 2: Rheumatoid arthritis (RA)				
Item 3: SLE and vasculitis				
Item 4: Acute multi-system connective tissue disease				
Item 5: Thrombosis and the antiphospholipid syndrome				
Item 6: Gout and pseudo-gout				
Item 7: Polymyalgia rheumatica/cranial arteritis				
Item 8: Acute back pain				
Item 9: Severe back pain/osteoporosis				
Item 10: Osteomyelitis				
Item 11: Septic arthritis				

	Learnt from practice	BLM used	SAQ completed	Other learning undertaken
Group 9 **Renal Disease**				
Item 1: Fluid balance and electrolytes: assessing fluid status				
Item 2: Fluid balance and electrolytes: sodium problems				
Item 3: Patient stopped passing urine				
Item 4: Left ventricular failure				
Item 5: Hyperkalaemia				
Item 6: The acidotic patient				
Item 7: Acute renal failure				
Item 8: Chronic renal failure				
Item 9: Multi-system vasculitis/acute glomerular nephritis				
Item 10: Intercurrent illness in dialysis and transplant patients				
Item 11: Nephrotic syndrome				
Group 10 **Cardiology**				
Item 1: Syncope				
Item 2: A clinical approach to patients with tachycardia				
Item 3: Atrial fibrillation				
Item 4: Bradycardia and pacing				
Item 5: Basic life support				
Item 6: Chest pain				
Item 7: Myocardial infarction – educating the patient				
Item 8: Myocardial infarction – heart failure and shock				
Item 9: Cardiogenic shock				
Item 10: Heart failure following a myocardial infarction				
Item 11: Myocardial infarction – secondary prevention				
Item 12: Post infarction arrhythmias				
Item 13: Acute myocardial ischaemia – who needs intervention?				
Item 14: Heart failure recognition and acute management				
Item 15: Aortic stenosis and other valvular heart disease				
Item 16: Infective endocarditis				
Item 17: Cor pulmonale				
Item 18: Cardiomyopathy				
Item 19: Investigating hypertension (HT)				
Item 20: Drug treatment of hypertension				
Item 21: The swollen/ischeamic leg				
Group 11 **Respiratory disorders**				
Item 1: Acute breathlessness				
Item 2: Cough				
Item 3: Breathlessness and wheeze				
Item 4: Hyperventilation				
Item 5: Haemoptysis				
Item 6: Chest pain				
Item 7: Respiratory failure				
Item 8: Chest X-rays				
Item 9: COPD – acute exacerbation				
Item 10: Pneumonia				
Item 11: Tuberculosis				
Item 12: Pleural effusion				
Item 13: Pulmonary embolism				
Item 14: Pneumothorax				
Item 15: Carcinoma of the bronchus				
Item 16: Sarcoidosis				

		Learnt from practice	BLM used	SAQ completed	Other learning undertaken
Group 12	**ITU**				
Item 1:	Shock				
Item 2:	Acute lung injury				
Group 13	**Poisoning**				
Item 1:	Self poisoning				
Item 2:	Paracetamol poisoning				
Item 3:	Salicylate, benzodiazepine and tricyclic antidepressant overdose				
Item 4:	Anaphylactic shock				
Group 14	**Endocrinology and diabetes**				
Item 1:	New diagnosis of diabetes mellitus				
Item 2:	Diabetic ketoacidosis				
Item 3:	Hyperosmolar non-ketotic coma				
Item 4:	Hypoglycaemic coma				
Item 5:	Sick diabetic patient				
Item 6:	Management of Type 2 diabetes mellitus				
Item 7:	Diabetic foot				
Item 8:	Urgent surgery in patients with diabetes				
Item 9:	Diabetes in pregnancy				
Item 10:	Emergency management of Cushing's syndrome				
Item 11:	Thyrotoxicosis				
Item 12:	Thyroid storm				
Item 13:	Amiodarone and thyroid function				
Item 14:	Hypothyroidism				
Item 15:	Difficult thyroid function tests				
Item 16:	Addison's disease				
Item 17:	Patients on steroids for surgery				
Item 18:	Incidental hypercalcaemia				
Item 19:	Severe hypercalcaemia				
Item 20:	Hypocalcaemia				
Item 21:	Phaeochromocytomas (Catecholamine crisis)				
Item 22:	Hypopituitary coma and apoplexy				
Item 23:	Diabetes insipidus				
Item 24:	The syndrome of inappropriate ADH (SIADH)				
Group 15	**Neurology**				
Item 1:	Diplopia				
Item 2:	Visual impairment or failure (acute/subacute)				
Item 3:	Bell's Palsy				
Item 4:	Vertigo				
Item 5:	Stroke and TIAs				
Item 6:	Subdural haemorrhage				
Item 7:	L-DOPA therapy				
Item 8:	Multiple sclerosis				
Item 9:	Encephalitis				
Item 10:	Falls				
Item 11:	Head injuries				
Item 12:	Meningitis				
Item 13:	Fits and faints				
Item 14:	Difficulty in walking				
Item 15:	Headaches				
Item 16:	Severe brain injury				
Item 17:	Movement disorders				

		Learnt from practice	BLM used	SAQ completed	Other learning undertaken
Group 16	**Psychiatry**				
Item 1:	Delirium				
Item 2:	Drugs and poisons as causes of delirium				
Item 3:	Dementia				
Item 4:	Delirium tremens (DT)				
Item 5:	Acute depression				
Item 6:	Suicide and deliberate self harm (DSH)				
Item 7:	Acute anxiety				
Item 8:	Opiate dependence				
Item 9:	Disturbed patient				
Group 17	**Dermatology**				
Item 1:	A swollen red leg				
Item 2:	Erythema nodosum				
Item 3:	Urticaria and angio-oedema				
Item 4:	Sun-induced rash				
Item 5:	Generalised rash or eruption				
Item 6:	Pruritus				
Item 7:	Cutaneous adverse drug reactions (ADR)				
Item 8:	HIV and the skin				

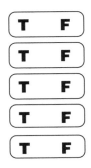

GROUP 1: Infectious diseases

Q1 In infection due to *Salmonella typhi*

a	Patients with infections due to *Salmonella typhi* usually have a peripheral leucocytosis	T F
b	Cefuroxine is the treatment of choice for typhoid	T F
c	*S. typhi* is an intracellular infection	T F
d	*S. typhi* is a zoonotic disease	T F
e	*S. typhi* is a notifiable disease	T F

Q2 In meningitis

a	A CT scan should always be performed in suspected cases of meningitis prior to doing a lumbar punture	T F
b	Septicaemia due to *N. meningitidis* has a higher mortality then meningococcal meningitis	T F
c	There is an effective vaccine for contacts of *N. meningitidis* Group B	T F
d	Rifampicin prophylaxis should be given to all medical and nursing staff contacts of patients with meningococcal meningitis	T F
e	Rifampicin can permanently stain soft contact lenses pink	T F

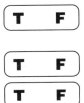

Q3 A trauma patient on the intensive care unit develops severe diarrhoea. Your consultant thinks that she may have developed pseudomembranous colitis

| a | What is the bacterial cause of pseudomembranous colitis?
How would you confirm the diagnosis? |

_____

_____

_____

| b | Briefly describe the pathophysiology of pseudomembranous colitis.
Which antibiotics are most commonly implicated in causing it? |

_____

_____

_____

c How would you manage the patient?

_____

_____

_____

Q4 In Varicella Zoster virus infection

a Chickenpox is more serious in children than in adults   T   F

b Varicella Zoster virus is the cause of both chickenpox and shingles   T   F

c A patient in hospital with shingles does not require isolation   T   F

d Shingles is due to reactivation of VZV in the dorsal root or cranial nerve ganglia   T   F

e Early treatment of shingles with aciclovir is thought to decrease the risk of patients developing post-herpetic neuralgia   T   F

f _Pseudomonas aeruginosa_ is the commonest cause of secondary bacterial infection in shingles   T   F

Q5 Regarding nosocomial infection

a Nosocomial (hospital acquired) bacteraemia is less common than community acquired bacteraemia   T   F

b Intravenous catheters are a common cause of nosocomial bacteraemia   T   F

c Ventilated patients are less likely to develop Gram negative sepsis secondary to respiratory tract infection than non-ventilated patients   T   F

d Nosocomial infections are increasingly a source of litigation in hospitals   T   F

e Respiratory tract infections are the commonest nosocomial infection   T   F

f Wound infections are the second commonest nosocomial infection   T   F

Q6 A 20-year-old female returns from a four-week backpacking trip around India and Nepal complaining of fever and malaise of two week duration. She turns up in your accident and emergency department and the casualty officer refers her to you as a case of PUO

a What is meant by the term PUO?

_____

_____

b

What questions should you ask returning travellers who present with fever?

_____

_____

_____

_____

_____

c

What initial investigations would you ask for?

_____

_____

_____

_____

d

Where would you nurse this patient assuming that she requires admisssion?

_____

_____

_____

_____

GROUP 2: STDs

Q1 In people infected with HIV

a *Mycobacterium tuberculosis* classically develops late in the course of infection while the patient is severely immunosuppressed   T   F

b Clinical infection due to *Mycobacterium tuberculosis* is frequently due to reactivation of dormant bacilli in a patient   T   F

c Presentation of infection due to *Mycobacterium tuberculosis* is often atypical   T   F

d Treatment of *Mycobacterium tuberculosis* can affect a patient's antiretroviral therapy   T   F

e Infections due to *Mycobacterium avium-intracellulare* complex become frequent once the CD4 lymphocyte count falls below 200/mm^3 T   F

Q2 In patients infected with HIV

a Pneumocystis pneumonia is usually of rapid onset   T   F

b Pneumocystis pneumonia is an AIDS defining illness   T   F

c Prophylaxis against *Pneumocystis carinii* should be given to patients with CD4 counts less than about 200/mm^3 T   F

d Bacterial infections, particularly with capsulated organisms are commoner than in the general population   T   F

e Bacterial respiratory tract infections usually have an insidious onset   T   F

GROUP 3: Nutrition

Q1 **Which of the following are the complications of parenteral nutrition?**

a	Hyperglycaemia	T	F
b	Cholestatic jaundice	T	F
c	Essential fatty acid deficiency	T	F
d	Pneumothorax	T	F
e	Raised plasma urea	T	F

Q2 **Which of the following statements for the sources of vitamins are correct?**

a	Vitamin A – liver	T	F
b	Folic acid – bread	T	F
c	Vitamin B12 – milk	T	F
d	Vitamin K – soya bean oil	T	F
e	Vitamin E – steak	T	F

Q3 **How do you ensure a positive nitrogen balance in a patient who is being fed enterally?**

_____

_____

_____

_____

_____

_____

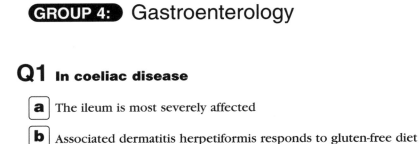

GROUP 4: Gastroenterology

Q1 In coeliac disease

a The ileum is most severely affected ⬚ T F

b Associated dermatitis herpetiformis responds to gluten-free diet ⬚ T F

c Oesophageal cancer is an associated complication ⬚ T F

d Measurement of B12 is a good screening test ⬚ T F

e Splenomegaly is a recognised association ⬚ T F

Q2 A 23-year-old beautician, who is otherwise well, complains of alternating diarrhoea, constipation and severe abdominal pain

a What are the possible causes?

_____

_____

b What investigations would you suggest?

_____

_____

c How would you manage the problem?

_____

_____

Q3 A 50-year-old man presents with dysphagia

a What are the possible causes?

_____

_____

b What questions in the history help you arrive at a diagnosis?

_____

_____

c What are the investigations to consider?

_____

_____

d If caused by cancer, how would you decide on treatment?

_____

_____

e What treatments are available for achalasia?

_____

_____

Q4 In a patient with diarrhoea

a A 24-hour stool weight of 200g suggests significant pathology   T   F

b Presence of blood makes an infective cause likely   T   F

c Measurement of a serum amylase is useful if pancreatic disease is suspected   T   F

d A normal sigmoidoscopy does not exclude colonic disease   T   F

e Antibiotics should be given if infection is suspected   T   F

Q5 A 30-year-old man presents with a 10 week history of discomfort in right iliac fossa. He has also noticed some weight loss. The ESR is also raised

a What is the differential diagnosis?

_____

_____

b How would you investigate him?

_____

_____

c Following confirmation of the diagnosis what treatment options are there?

_____

_____

Q6 **An elderly gentleman collapses following the passage of a large amount of blood PR late one evening**

a What are the most likely causes of this?

_____

_____

b His blood pressure is 80/60 and pulse rate 120. How would you manage him?

_____

_____

c How would you establish a cause?

_____

_____

Q7 **A 40-year-old woman complains of fatigue and lethargy. You notice her Hb to be low at 8 g/dl.**

a A low MCV indicates iron deficiency and endoscopy should be performed as the next test   T   F

b In iron deficiency the serum iron, TIBC and ferritin will be reduced   T   F

c Faecal occult blood tests do not contribute to the diagnosis   T   F

d A history of terminal ileal resection suggests macrocytic anaemia due to folate deficiency as a possible cause   T   F

e If there are no other symptoms menorrhagia is the likeliest cause   T   F

Q8 A 55-year-old man presents with a two-month history of epigastric pain

a If peptic ulceration is suspected clinically a therapeutic trial of a proton pump inhibitor is appropriate
T   F

b A normal serum amylase makes a pancreatic disorder unlikely
T   F

c As he has had numerous courses of treatment from his GP a blood test for HP aetiology should be performed to check his HP status before commencing treatment
T   F

d Following a normal endoscopy, eradication of helicobacter is unlikely to help his symptoms
T   F

e Once the *H.pylori* is successfully eradicated the recurrence rate is less than 1 per cent per annum, in the UK
T   F

GROUP 5: Liver, biliary and pancreatic disorders

Q1 A 70-year-old presents with a swollen abdomen and shifting dullness. He has no history of previous illnesses

a What is the differential diagnosis?

_____
_____
_____
_____

b What investigations should be performed?

_____
_____
_____
_____

c What treatments are indicated?

_____
_____
_____
_____
_____

Q2 A 48-year-old obese female presents to A&E deeply jaundiced, confused and disorientated

a A common bile duct stone is the common cause of this form of jaundice   T   F

b N-Acetyl cysteine should be considered even without knowledge of toxicology results   T   F

c Insulin is frequently required to treat the hyperglycaemia associated with her liver failure   T   F

d Laxatives are indicated to clear her bowel of protein   T   F

e Liver transplant is contraindicated in fulminant viral hepatitis because of the risk of immunosuppression.   T   F

Q3 **A 65-year-old known alcoholic is admitted following a bout of vomiting copious bright red blood. He had 'veins' injected in his oesophagus 3 years ago**

a One should assume he has bleeding oesophageal varices and commence appropriate pharmacological therapy immediately 　　　T　　F

b Endoscopic injection of dilute adrenaline into the varix is the treatment of choice for varices 　　T　　F

c TIPPS should be considered if bleeding gastric varices are discovered 　　T　　F

d Long term pharmacological therapy has no role in the management of oesophageal varices 　　T　　F

e Banding of oesophageal varies is preferable to injection sclerotherapy 　　T　　F

Q4 **A 62-year-old female, who was previously well, is referred by her GP with an ALT 120, AST 200, Alk phos 400. An ultrasound of her abdomen reveals a slightly enlarged liver, moderate splenomegaly but no other abnormality**

a What are the possible causes of the abnormal LFTs?

_____

_____

_____

_____

b Her investigations revealed that her viral markers are negative but her ANA is positive at a titre of 1/80 and AMA positive of 1/120. What do these results suggest and how would you clarify the diagnosis?

_____

_____

_____

_____

c Once the diagnosis is established what further investigations or treatment should be considered?

_____

_____

_____

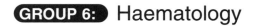

GROUP 6: Haematology

Q1 In a patient with a microcytic anaemia, the following laboratory tests are used to confirm a diagnosis of iron deficiency

a	Serum iron	T F
b	HbA_2	T F
c	Serum ferritin	T F
d	Serum erythropoietin	T F
e	Serum transferrin receptor	T F

Q2 In patients with confirmed pernicious anaemia indicate whether the following statements are true or false

a	The blood count at diagnosis will show a macrocytic anaemia	T F
b	Gastric parietal cell antibodies are positive	T F
c	Malabsorption of ^{57}Co-vitamin B_{12} is corrected by the addition of porcine intrinsic factor	T F
d	The haemoglobin concentration reaches higher levels at a faster rate if three injections of 1000µg hydroxocobalamin IM are given at 3 day intervals	T F
e	Little is to be gained by further blood tests once treatment has been initiated	T F

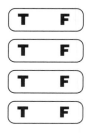

Q3 A 35-year-old woman with four children is admitted for an elective cholecystectomy. Surgery is uneventful but three days post operatively she is noted to have a haemoglobin concentration of 8.9g/dl. The haemoglobin was normal previously. She is transfused two units of plasma reduced blood and discharged home. She presents to the A&E department seven days after discharge with the recent onset of widespread bruising, epistaxis and headache. A coagulation screen was normal but she has severe thrombocytopenia

Hb 11.2 g/dl

MCV 84 fl

WBC 12.2 x10^9/$_1$

Platelets 5 x10^9/$_1$

PT/INR 12 secs /1.0 PTTK 32 secs.

Fibrinogen 4.6 g/l

a What is the likely cause of her thrombocytopenia?

_____
_____

b Should she receive a transfusion of platelets?

_____
_____

c What other therapeutic measures might be helpful?

_____
_____

d What should you tell the patient?

_____
_____

Q4 **A 47-year-old Afro-Caribbean woman was started on treatment with carbimazole for hyperthyroidism. She presents with a sore throat, as she was told to do, two weeks after starting treatment. She is pyrexial (38.4°C) with injected fauces but no oral ulceration. A blood count indicates neutropenia but no other abnormality**

Hb 12.4 g/dl

MCV 89fl

WBC 1.9 x10^9/l

Neutrophils 0.8 x x10^9/l

Lymphocytes 0.7 x10^9/l

Monocytes 0.3 x10^9/l

Eosinophils 0.1 x10^9/l

Platelets 260 x10^9/l

a Give four possible causes for her neutropenia

1 _____

2 _____

3 _____

4 _____

b What would be your immediate management?

_____

_____

Q5 Regarding blood transfusion

a In an emergency, the transfusion of group O Rh(D) negative blood is appropriate and safe   **T**   **F**

b The commonest cause of a serious haemolytic transfusion reaction is failure to identify a red cell antibody on laboratory screening   **T**   **F**

c A formula, such as 2 units of FFP per 5 units of blood, is the correct way to manage blood product support during a massive blood transfusion   **T**   **F**

d Patients who have repeated blood transfusions and recurrent febrile transfusion reactions should receive prophylactic hydrocortisone and chlorpheniramine prior to each transfusion   **T**   **F**

Q6 A 56-year-old woman presents to casualty with a nose bleed which had continued for two hours despite simple measures. She has had several such episodes over the last two months, and is noted to have widespread purpura. Her only other complaint is of night time cramps in the legs. She is febrile (38.2°C) with signs and symptoms of an URTI and admits to long standing excess alcohol consumption. A spleen is palpable just below the costal margin. A blood count confirms the clinical impression of thrombocytopenia

Hb 11.1 g/dl

MCV 106 fl

WBC 3.4 x10^9/l

Platelets 10 x10^9/l

a Suggest six possible reasons for this patient's thrombocytopenia

_____

_____

_____

_____

_____

_____

_____

_____

b She undergoes bone marrow aspiration. Tick the following features of the bone marrow which would be compatible with a diagnosis of ITP

Hypercellular

Increased numbers of megakaryocytes

More than 10% blast cells

Normal erythroid and granulocyte maturation

Micromegakaryocytes

Megaloblastic erythropoiesis

c There is no history of quinine ingestion and folate levels are normal. Bone marrow examination together with the severity of thrombocytopenia support a diagnosis of ITP. List the causes of immune platelet destruction

_____

_____

_____

_____

_____

_____

d This patient had a positive ANA with increased IgG and IgM anticardiolipin antibodies. A coagulation screen showed an APTT of 61 secs but was otherwise normal. What is the likely cause of the prolonged APTT?

_____

_____

_____

_____

e The patient has SLE with secondary ITP and anti-phospholipid antibodies. Bleeding is related to the thrombocytopenia; lupus anti-coagulants are associated paradoxically with arterial or venous thrombosis. What measures would you take to control this patient's bleeding?

_____

_____

Q7 **Continued or recurrent bleeding after surgery is a common problem. It is important to distinguish between surgical blood loss and failure of the haemostatic system as soon as possible. Which of the following observations would suggest that blood loss is related to impaired haemostasis?**

Acute, dramatic presentation ☐

Associated renal or liver disease ☐

Bleeding from the surgical site only ☐

Persistent, prolonged bleeding ☐

The presence of purpura and oozing from venepuncture sites ☐

Rate of blood loss requiring transfusion in excess of 4 units/hour ☐

Q8 **Surgical bleeding and impaired haemostasis can co-exist and prolonged surgical blood loss requiring large volume blood transfusion will itself result in a haemostatic defect due to dilution or DIC. Haemostatic failure post-operatively is usually due to an acquired defect, although mild, inherited disorders of coagulation may not present until haemostatic challenge in adult life**

a Which of the following laboratory abnormalities would suggest an inherited defect of coagulation?

Prolonged PT and APTT ☐

Isolated decrease in the fibrinogen concentration ☐

Increased fibrin D-dimers ☐

Isolated increase in the APTT which fails to correct on the addition of normal plasma in vitro ☐

Isolated increase in the PT ☐

b What does an increase in fibrin D-dimers imply? ☐

_____

_____

c Under what circumstances would the concentration of fibrin D-dimers increase?

_____

_____

Q9 **Failure of a prolonged APTT to correct with the addition of normal plasma in vitro suggests an acquired inhibitor of coagulation rather than a factor deficiency.**

Name three inhibitors of coagulation in order of the frequency encountered

1 _____

2 _____

3 _____

Q10 **A ten-year-old Nigerian boy presents to casualty. His parents tell you that he has sickle cell anaemia and has just arrived in the UK. He speaks little English, is febrile and looks frightened but is lying quietly on the bed and does not appear to be in severe pain**

a How would you establish the diagnosis of HbSS?

b Physical examination reveals icteric sclerae, a pansystolic murmur and a palpable spleen, but no bony tenderness or swelling. Which of these features are to be expected in a patient with sickle cell anaemia?

c Icteric sclerae   [   ]

Pansystolic murmur   [   ]

Palpable spleen   [   ]

Bony tenderness   [   ]

Swelling   [   ]

d In the absence of any evidence of a painful sickle cell crisis, should this patient be sent home?

Give three possible reasons for splenomegaly in this child?

1 _____

2 _____

3 _____

e A blood count showed

Hb	4.6g/dl
MCV	78 fl
WBC	15.6 x10^9/l
Platelets	60 x10^9/l
Reticulocytes	5.1%

In what way does the FBC differ from that expected in a patient with sickle cell anaemia?

_____

_____

f The results of the FBC together with the fever suggests infection with suppression of bone marrow activity. Splenic sequestration sufficient to cause a fall in the haemoglobin concentration to this degree would have been accompanied by signs of hypovolaemia. In addition to malaria, parvovirus B19 should be excluded. This virus specifically infects RBC precursors and results in a fall in Hb concentration and reticulocytopenia in patients with a chronic haemolytic anaemia. The laboratory reports that there are malaria parasites on the blood film. What other information do you need?

_____

_____

_____

_____

g This patient had Plasmodium falciparum malaria with a parasitaemia of 3.2% and ring trophozoites only seen on blood film review. Repeated malaria infections are likely to be the reason for his splenomegaly. Give four reasons why this patient's anaemia may have been made worse by inter-current infection with malaria?

1 _____

2 _____

3 _____

4 _____

h Explain why this child has malaria when the sickle cell mutation is said to protect against malaria

_____

_____

Q11 **A 40-year-old female underwent mitral valve replacement for rheumatic mitral valve disease. Post-operatively she was placed on warfarin anti-coagulation to prevent valve thrombosis**

a For how long should anticoagulation continue?

Six months   [   ]

Three years   [   ]

Life-long   [   ]

b What is the target INR?

_____

c What is the INR and how is it derived?

_____

_____

_____

_____

d The patient was referred to the local anticoagulant clinic and seen initially on a weekly basis with warfarin dose adjustment until the INR was stable in the therapeutic stage.
Give four common reasons for loss of anticoagulant control in patients taking warfarin?

1 _____

2 _____

3 _____

4 _____

e Stable anticoagulation was achieved with an INR of 3.2-3.9 on 6mg of warfin daily. Nine months later, following investigation for a persistent cough, a diagnosis of pulmonary TB was made and anti-tuberculous chemotherapy was started with isoniazid, rifampicin and pyrazinamide. How would you expect anticoagulant control to be affected by this and what action would you take?

_____

_____

_____

f A stable INR on a higher dose of warfarin was achieved, on average 8.5-10mg daily. Five months later the patient was well and went to visit her sister in Australia. She was warned to register with an anti-coagulant clinic there and continue regular monitoring. Two months later she was admitted as an emergency to a hospital in Australia with a short history of confusion and disorientation. A CT scan showed a large subdural haematoma; the INR on admission was 7.0. Why had anti-coagulant control been lost?

_____

_____

_____

g Shortly after admission, focal-neurological signs developed and a further CT scan demonstrated intra-cerebral haemorrhage. What is the most appropriate way of reversing anti-coagulation prior to emergency surgery?

10mg vitamin K IV

10mg vitamin K IV plus two units (500ml) FFP

5mg vitamin K IV plus prothrombin complex concentrate (50u/kg)

0.5mg vitamin K IV plus four units (1.0L) FFP

h Why is the dose of vitamin K important?

Q12 List three causes for anaemia in myeloma

1

2

3

Q13 A patient with an elevated Hb is more likely to have secondary polycythaemia than polycythaemia vera if

a Splenomegaly is absent   T   F

b Red cell mass is normal   T   F

c The platelet count is normal   T   F

d The patient has Down's syndrome   T   F

e Serum urate level is raised   T   F

Q14 Characteristic features of low grade lymphoma include

a Leucocytosis   T   F

b Long survival   T   F

c Cure rate of 25%   T   F

d Haemolytic anaemia   T   F

e Diagnostic chromosomal abnormalities in 50% of cases   T   F

Q15 The following are characteristic associations

a Acute lymphoblastic leukaemia and t(15;17) translocation   T   F

b Chronic myeloid leukaemia and gout   T   F

c Myelodysplastic syndrome and paraproteinaemia   T   F

d Alkylating agents and secondary leukaemias   T   F

e Complex karyotypic abnormalities in acute leukaemia and prolonged survival   T   F

Q16 A 24-year-old woman complaining of tiredness was found to have Hb 9.8g/dl. Her GP could palpate small glands in both groins and was worried that the patient might have acute leukaemia. Outline your assessment of the patient that would confirm or exclude the diagnosis

_____

_____

_____

_____

Q17 A 62-year-old man with a platelet count of 840 x10^9/l is likely to have a reactive thrombocytosis rather than essential thrombocythaemia if

a His WBC is 20 x10^9/l   T   F

b The spleen is palpable   T   F

c No karyotypic abnormalities are found in the marrow   T   F

d He has burning discomfort in his hands and feet   T   F

e He is iron deficient   T   F

Q18 Say whether the following statements about a high white cell count are true or false

a Peripheral blood eosinophilia may be seen in patients receiving corticosteroids   T   F

b Lymphocytosis is a feature of pertussis infection   T   F

c In neutrophilia, toxic granulation confirms an infective cause   T   F

d Leucostasis due to WCC of 200 x10^9/l is best treated with cytoreductive chemotherapy   T   F

e Leucocytosis is common following splenectomy   T   F

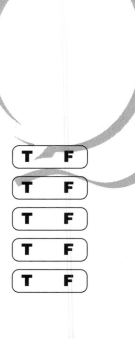

Q19 A normal MCV is found in

a Patient following a brisk upper GIT bleed   **T**   **F**

b ß thalassaemia trait   **T**   **F**

c Sickle cell anaemia (HbSS)   **T**   **F**

d Folate deficiency   **T**   **F**

e Chronic alcoholism   **T**   **F**

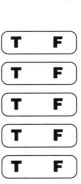

GROUP 7: Geriatrics

Q1 What are the main components of a discharge plan for elderly patients?

_____

_____

_____

_____

Q2 The following drugs are commonly associated with _C. difficile infection_

a	Amoxicillin	T	F
b	Erythromycin	T	F
c	Clindamycin	T	F
d	Vancomycin	T	F
e	Metronidazole	T	F

Q3 Amiodarone

a	Can cause hypothyroidism	T	F
b	Can cause hyperthyroidism	T	F
c	Has negative inotopic effect	T	F
d	May cause deranged LFT	T	F
e	May cause corneal deposits	T	F

Q4 Non-steroidal anti inflammatory agents

a	Are a common cause of upper GIT bleeding and iron deficiency anaemia in the elderly	T	F
b	Their effect on gastric mucosa can be significantly minimised by H2-antagonists	T	F
c	May worsen heart failure because of fluid retention	T	F
d	Their effect on gastric mucosa can be minimised by corticosteroids	T	F
e	May cause confusion in the elderly	T	F

Q5 A 79-year-old man was brought into A&E by his wife with his third fall in a month. He had extensive bruising and a laceration on his occiput. He had left hip pain on standing and denied loss of consciousness

a What further information would you seek about the fall?

_____

_____

_____

_____

b What investigations would you perform and why?

_____

_____

_____

_____

c ECG shows slow AF at a rate of 45bpm. How could you manage him now?

_____

_____

_____

_____

Q6 Are the following statements about orthostatic hypotension (OH) true or false?

a Antihypertensive drugs can cause OH   T   F

b OH is always caused by drugs   T   F

c Patients with OH should avoid caffeine containing drinks   T   F

d Cardiac pacing helps symptoms of OH   T   F

e Chest infection can cause OH   T   F

Q7 The following would support a diagnosis of epilepsy as a cause for blackout in the elderly:

a Post blackout dysphasia   T   F

b Incontinence   T   F

c Pallor observed during blackout   T   F

d Normal ECG   T   F

e Small vessel disease on CT scan   T   F

Q8 An 85-year-old man with non insulin dependent diabetes mellitus (Type 2) was admitted with chest pain. His ECG shows an acute anterior MI. A CXR shows upper lobe blood diversion. He has crackles at both bases on examination. The JVP is not raised and his BP is 110/60

a What further history would you take?

_____

_____

_____

_____

b What treatment would you institute?

_____

_____

_____

_____

c His pain settles and he has no dysrrhythmia in the first 24 hours. Do you add any therapy on the post take ward round?

_____

_____

_____

_____

_____

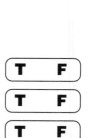

Q9 When making a diagnosis of delirium the following are important

a	Acute onset	T F
b	Normal level of consciousness	T F
c	Presence of consolidation in chest examination	T F
d	Female sex	T F
e	Poor short term memory	T F

Q10 List four causes of delirium

1 _____

2 _____

3 _____

4 _____

Q11 Which of the following statements on depression are true?

a	May present with dementia	T F
b	For diagnosis high score on Geriatric Depression Scale is essential	T F
c	Hypothyroidism may present with depression	T F
d	Suicidal thoughts/intent warrants referral to a psychiatrist	T F

Q12 Are the following statements about dementia true or false?

a	The incidence increases with age	T F
b	Firm diagnosis can be made as a result of MMSE assessment	T F
c	All patients with dementia of Alzheimer's type improve on an acetyl choline transferase inhibitor such as donepezil	T F
d	Is a risk factor for delirium	T F
e	Lewy-body dementia patients are more susceptible to side-effects of anti-psychotic drugs	T F

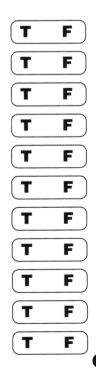

Q13 **List four treatable conditions that may present with dementia-like illness**

1 _____

2 _____

3 _____

4 _____

Q14 **A 79-year-old man is brought to A&E by his niece with a three day history of confusion and falls. On examination he has coarse crackles at the left base. Which of the following would be helpful in making the diagnosis?**

a History from GP   T   F

b Drug history   T   F

c Assessment using Abbreviated Mental Test score   T   F

d Assessment using Geriatric Depression Score   T   F

e CT scan of head   T   F

f Chest X-ray   T   F

g MSU   T   F

Q15 **Known aetiological factors and associated clinical conditions for hypothermia include**

a Antidepressants   T   F

b Phenothiazine   T   F

c Hypothyroidism   T   F

d Thyrotoxicosis   T   F

e Non-steroidal anti-inflammatory drugs   T   F

f Parkinsonism   T   F

g Diabetes mellitus   T   F

h Increased shivering   T   F

i Impaired temperature perception   T   F

j Reduced heat production   T   F

k Impaired thermoregulation   T   F

Q16 Clinical manifestation of hypothermia include

a	Confusion	T	F
b	Impaired conscious level	T	F
c	Prolonged PR interval	T	F
d	'J' waves on ECG in all patients	T	F
e	Neck stiffness in patients will severe hypothermia	T	F

Q17 Complications of hypothermia include

a	Pancreatitis	T	F
b	Oliguria	T	F
c	Ventricular fibrillation	T	F
d	Vascular thromboses	T	F

Q18 Patients with hypothermia should have urgent

a	Blood glucose	T	F
b	ECG	T	F
c	Urea and electrolytes	T	F
d	Chest X-rays	T	F
e	Blood gases	T	F
f	Cortisol level	T	F
g	TFTs	T	F
h	Serum amylase	T	F

Q19 An 89-year-old retired teacher is referred for assessment with a 3 day history of immobility following 2 falls and incontinence of urine. On examination she is acutely confused with AMT score of 5/10. Physical examination is normal and in particular she has no temperature.

a What initial investigations would you perform?

_____

_____

_____

b Results of initial investigations come back normal apart from urine which has revealed ++protein and ++blood on dipstick and MSU growth of *E. Coli*, 10^5/ml.

What is the cause of her falls/confusion?

_____

_____

_____

c Three days after admission she collapses while walking with a physiotherapist. On examination she had tachycardia (110 regular and BP of 110/70 mmHg). ECG revealed deep T wave inversion in all chest leads. When questioned the patient stated that she felt 'giddy' before collapsing and did not have any chest pain. What is the cause of her collapse?

_____

_____

_____

_____

Q20 **Match the scale with parameter to be measured**

a Barthel scale ☐

b Mini-Mental State examination ☐

c Geriatric Depression scale ☐

d Waterlow score ☐

e Philadelphia Geriatric Morale scale ☐

1 Quality of life

2 Cognition

3 Pressure sore risk

4 Activities of Daily Living

5 Depression

Q21 **List the main risk factors for stroke**

_____

_____

_____

_____

_____

Q22 **List three possible sources of embolism in ischaemic stroke**

1 _____

2 _____

3 _____

Q23 **Most strokes occur in the vertebro-basilar territory** (T   F)

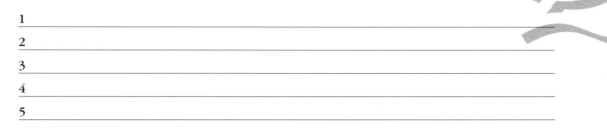

Q24 **List five conditions which might present like acute stroke**

1 _____

2 _____

3 _____

4 _____

5 _____

Q25 **List the most important early complications of stroke**

_____

_____

_____

_____

_____

Q26 **Aspirin is the only available treatment for secondary prevention of stroke**   [T   F]

Q27 **Carotid endarterectomy should be offered to all patients having multiple TIAs**   [T   F]

Q28 **What factors are considered important in DNR decision making? List them below**

_____

_____

_____

_____

_____

_____

Q29 **Are the following statements relating to Parkinsonism true or false?**

a Tremor occurs in all patients with Parkinson's disease   T   F

b A history of hypertension makes the diagnosis of arteriosclerotic Parkinsonism more likely   T   F

c Drug induced Parkinsonism is most often caused by antidepressants   T   F

d A CT scan will confirm a patient has Parkinson's Disease   T   F

Q30 **List five causes of an acutely ca swollen joint**

1 _____

2 _____

3 _____

4 _____

5 _____

Q31 **Gout is the commonest cause of an acute hot joint in elderly people?**   T   F

Q32 **List the important investigations when managing a patient with an acute hot joint**

_____

_____

_____

_____

_____

_____

Q33 The following are treatments for the hot joint

a Diclofenac and misoprostol

b Aspirin

c Prednisolone

d Methyl prednisolone injections

e Allopurinol

f Aminophylline

g Colchicine

h Lignocaine injection

i Nalidixic acid

j Flucloxacillin

k Gentamicin

l Indomethacin

m Benzyl penicillin

Q34 For each patient (below), select the most appropriate treatment/ treatments in the acute situation from the list above. Each option may be used once, more than once or not at all

a A 75-year-old man with severe heart failure on high dose diuretics presents with an acutely swollen ankle. The serum uric acid is 600µmol/l

_____

_____

b A 68-year-old lady with chronic arthritis presents with a painful swollen knee. Joint aspiration reveals negatively birefringent crystals

_____

_____

c A 78-year-old lady with chronic rheumatoid arthritis presents with a hot swollen elbow. She is pyrexial at 38.8°C and has a raised WCC

_____

_____

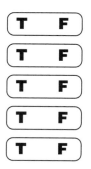

Q34 Pyrophosphate crystals are positively birefringent under polarised light?

T   F

Q35 Regarding pressure sores, mean capillary pressure in an adult is 100mmHg?

T   F

Q36 List four groups of patients at risk of developing pressure sores

1 _____

2 _____

3 _____

4 _____

Q37 List the reasons for grading pressure sores

_____

_____

_____

_____

_____

Q38 Important investigations when assessing a patient with a pressure sore include

a Haemoglobin   T   F

b Albumin   T   F

c Alkaline phosphatase   T   F

d Calcium   T   F

e Blood glucose   T   F

Q39 List the important risk factors in the development of pressure sores

_____

_____

_____

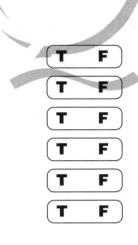

Q40 The following drugs may delay wound healing

a Metronidazole		T F
b Prednisolone		T F
c Calcium		T F
d Zinc		T F
e Naproxen		T F
f Aspirin		T F

Q41 What is the reason for X-raying the underlying bone in a long-standing pressure sore?

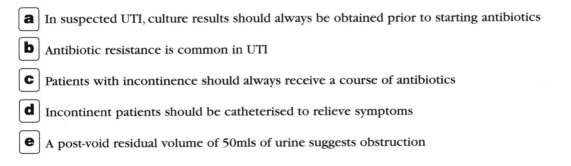

Q42 Regarding heart disease in the elderly

a Patients with severe dementia should not receive anticoagulation in AF	T F
b Anticoagulation is of no benefit in patients over 75 in AF	T F
c Acute MI may be silent in up to 10% of elderly patients	T F
d Elderly patients with heart failure should not receive ACE inhibition	T F
e β blockers are poorly tolerated in the elderly	T F

Q43 Regarding urinary problems in the elderly

a In suspected UTI, culture results should always be obtained prior to starting antibiotics	T F
b Antibiotic resistance is common in UTI	T F
c Patients with incontinence should always receive a course of antibiotics	T F
d Incontinent patients should be catheterised to relieve symptoms	T F
e A post-void residual volume of 50mls of urine suggests obstruction	T F

Q44 A 90-year-old woman with long-standing dementia reattends A&E after recent discharge, after a four week admission following a minor stroke. She had been discharged with two times daily homecare for washing and dressing, as well as meals-on-wheels daily. Since discharge a week ago, she had phoned 999 twice due to loneliness, and had been found by her homecarers to have left the front door open overnight. She had not eaten meals-on-wheels regularly.

a What are your priorities in A&E?

_____

_____

_____

_____

_____

_____

b Her mental test score (abbreviated) is 5/10, and her old notes show that she is in the same physical, mental and functional state as when she left hospital.

Which of the following would you do?

Admit her and transfer her back to the discharging team the next morning ⬭

Discharge her back home ⬭

Phone duty social worker ⬭

GROUP 8: Rheumatology

Q1 The following conditions are in the group of diseases known as the seronegative spondyloarthropathies

a	Enteropathic arthritis (ulcerative colitis/Crohn's)	T F
b	Reiter's syndrome	T F
c	Psoriatic arthritis	T F
d	Calcium pyrophosphate arthropathy	T F
e	Pott's disease of the spine	T F

Q2 In rheumatoid arthritis

a	Ulnar deviation is an early manifestation	T F
b	Vertical subluxation may occur at the atlantoaxial joint	T F
c	Disease modifying agents are only used after erosions develop	T F
d	The absence of IgM anti IgG rheumatoid factor excludes RA	T F
e	Carpal tunnel syndrome may be a presenting feature	T F

Q3 In psoriatic arthropathy

a	HLA B27 positivity is associated with spondylitis	T F
b	Arthritis mutilans is the most common pattern	T F
c	Onychopathy (nail pitting, ridging or onycholysis) is frequently associated with disease of the adjacent DIP joint	T F
d	The severity and extent of synovitis is proportional to the extent of the psoriasis	T F
e	Sulphasalazine may improve both psoriasis and arthritis	T F

Q4 In Wegener's granulomatosis

a Arthralgia is seen in more than 50 per cent of patients   T   F

b pANCA (perinuclear staining antineutrophil cytoplasmic antibody) is diagnostic   T   F

c Sinusitis is almost universally seen   T   F

d Mononeuritis multiplex may be a feature   T   F

e The treatment of choice is corticosteroids alone   T   F

Q5 In classical polyarteritis nodosa

a Hepatitis B may be positive in 10 per cent of patients   T   F

b Pulmonary haemorrhage is seen in 30 per cent of patients   T   F

c Renal infarction may occur   T   F

d Peripheral neuropathy occurs in 50 per cent of patients   T   F

e Necrotising crescentic glomerulonephritis is common   T   F

Q6 In systemic lupus erythematosus

a Lupus profundus is a common complication   T   F

b Renal vein thrombosis may occur   T   F

c The diagnosis of cerebral involvement can be confirmed by CSF examination   T   F

d Anti Sm antibodies are specific   T   F

e Anti Ro and anti La antibodies increase the risk of neonatal lupus syndrome   T   F

Q7 An elderly man presents with a swollen knee. The following are likely possibilities

a Early onset rheumatoid arthritis   T   F

b Pseudogout   T   F

c Gout   T   F

d Osteomalacia   T   ·F

e Osteoporosis   T   F

Q8 In primary Sjögren's syndrome

a Minor salivary gland biopsy showing absent lymphocytic infiltration is diagnostic   T F

b Schirmer's test is useful   T F

c Mononeuritis multiplex may occur   T F

d Cryoglobulinaemic vasculitis may be seen   T F

e The absence of anti-Ro antibodies excludes the diagnosis   T F

Q9 In a woman with primary nodal generalised osteoarthritis

a Involvement of the radiocarpal joint is characteristic   T F

b There is often a family history   T F

c Osler's nodes are characteristic   T F

d Vertebral osteoporosis is very common   T F

e Involvement of the metacarpophalangeal joint is common   T F

Q10 In acute lumbar disc prolapse

a Absolute bed rest is mandatory   T F

b A negative Lasègue's test excludes the diagnosis   T F

c Schmorl's nodes may be seen radiologically   T F

d The L 2/3 disc is the commonest level   T F

e Usually requires an MRI scan to visualise the disc lesion   T F

Q11 Polymyalgia rheumatica

a Usually presents acutely   T F

b May lead to the development of rheumatoid arthritis   T F

c May respond rapidly to an intramuscular injection of methylprednisolone 120 mg stat   T F

d May involve shoulder effusions   T F

e Has myelomatosis as a differential diagnosis   T F

Q12 In osteoporosis

a Previous oral contraceptive use is protective   T   F

b Moderate alcohol intake is protective   T   F

c Thyrotoxicosis may predispose to osteoporosis   T   F

d Fracture risk is related to T scores on DEXA   T   F

e Colles fractures are a characteristic presenting injury   T   F

Q13 In ANCA positive vasculitis

a Rapidly progressive necrotising glomerulonephritis is characteristic   T   F

b Pulmonary renal syndromes may occur   T   F

c cANCA has specificity for proteinase 3   T   F

d Necrotising alveolar capillaritis may lead to pulmonary haemorrhage   T   F

e Corneal melting may occur   T   F

Q14 Write short notes on the main clinical features of systemic sclerosis

_____

_____

_____

_____

_____

_____

_____

_____

_____

_____

_____

_____

_____

GROUP 9: Renal

Q1 **A 72-year-old man with a past history of smoking, hypertension and intermittent claudication presented with sudden onset of dyspnoea. He was peripherally cool with bilateral coarse crackles in his chest and bilateral pitting oedema to the knees.**

a What are the causes of systemic peripheral vascular shut-down?

_____

_____

b What clinical signs would indicate that there could be intravascular fluid overload?

_____

_____

c What is the implication (in terms of fluid status) of his peripheral oedema?

_____

_____

d On examination, he had signs of intravascular fluid overload and CXR showed pulmonary oedema. What physical signs would you look for before starting him on an ACE inhibitor?

_____

_____

e If you were concerned that he might have renal artery stenosis (RAS), what imaging of his kidneys would you do first?

_____

_____

f What findings on imaging would make the diagnosis of RAS more likely?

_____

_____

Q2 **You have been asked to review a 60-year-old man who was admitted 2 weeks ago with pneumonia. Despite IV ceftriaxone he has remained febrile with elevated ESR and CRP and an unexplained platelet count of 487. His creatinine was 124 on admission, but has now risen to 360. His Hb was 10.3. On examination he is cool peripherally with a BP of 120/70 lying and 85/60 standing.**

a Give 2 possible causes of his deterioration in renal function

1 _____

2 _____

b What bedside test would help in investigating the cause of his renal failure?

_____

_____

c What specific findings on examination or at the bedside would support each of your differential renal diagnoses?

_____

_____

d The next day after being given 2L saline and 1L of starch-based colloid he became acutely unwell, SOB and confused with a BP of 90/60. His Hb had fallen to 7.3gm/dL and creatinine had risen to 420. CXR shows extension of shadowing from the left base (at presentation) to involve both middle and lower zones. What do you think has happened?

_____

_____

e Outline your further management

_____

_____

_____

_____

Q3 **You have a patient with renal failure of unknown cause. He is anuric**

a What practical procedure should be performed first?

_____

b What must you consider if the bladder is empty?

_____

_____

Q4 **A routine pre-operative patient has a serum Na+ of 120 mmol/l. The patient is asymptomatic**

a How can you correct this in time for surgery tomorrow?

_____

_____

What should be your first action?

b

_____

_____

What is your initial recommendation?

c _____

_____

Q5 **A patient has a diagnosis of CRF and presents with an acute deterioration in renal function. He is vomiting**

a What must you do first?

_____

_____

b What future management is useful?

_____

_____

GROUP 10: Cardiology

Q1 **A 26-year-old man presents with a narrow complex tachycardia with rate of 194.**

a What immediate treatment is appropriate? (tick more than one if you wish)

Intravenous digoxin

Intravenous amiodarone

DC cardioversion

Supine valsalva manoeuvre

Intravenous adenosine

b The patient responds to your immediate treatment and the ECG in sinus rhythm shows a short PR interval with delta waves. The patient should be (tick all that apply)

Referred for 24 hour tape

Referred for electrophysiological study

Given long term oral digoxin

Given long term oral amiodarone

Referred for echocardiogram

Q2 **The following may be used when investigating hypertension**

ECG	Renal ultrasound
FBC	LFT
Urinary cortisol excretion	Intravenous pyelogram
Urinary sodium excretion	Urea + electrolytes
CXR	CT scan abdomen
Plasma renin/aldosterone	MIBG
Isotope renogram	Echocardiogram
Urinary catecholamines	

List the preferred order of investigations in the following patients

a A 22-year-old girl with a BP of 150/100 on oral contraceptive pill. She is overweight with negative FH and no positive finding

_____

_____

b A 48-year-old executive found to have BP 180/110 on insurance medical. Positive FH. Plethoric appearance. No CV findings

_____

_____

c A 68-year-old diabetic with BP 180/80 despite treatment with enalapril and hydrochlorothiazide. Electrolytes normal but urea 15.6 mmol/l (creatinine 212 mmol/l)

_____

_____

d A 38-year-old man recently saw his GP with palpitations and anxiety and had a BP of 160/110. Thyroid function tests normal but serum K^+ 2.9 mmol/l

_____

_____

Q3 The following may be used in treating cardiac failure

IV diuretic	Beta blocker
Oral nitrate	IV diamorphine
Oral digoxin	Oral ACEI
IV ACEI	Buccal nitrate
IV nitrate	Oral diuretic
IV digoxin	IV frusemide

What is your preferred therapeutic route in a 76-year-old man with a rapid irregular pulse and signs of pulmonary oedema?

_____

_____

_____

_____

Q4 A 56-year-old woman is admitted with severe chest pain that has persisted for 90 minutes

a Name the most likely diagnoses in order of importance

b What 4 questions would you use to differentiate the diagnoses?

1 _____

2 _____

3 _____

4 _____

c What are the first three tests you would choose if you suspect dissection?

1 _____

2 _____

3 _____

Q5 A 64-year-old man who had CABG 10 years ago, is brought to casualty after collapsing at home. He appears pale and sweating but is free from pain; nurses record a pulse of 140+ and a BP of 90 systolic. The ECG shows a regular broad complex tachycardia

a What is your immediate management?

_____

_____

b The patient reverts to sinus rhythm with the lignocaine bolus and the resting ECG shows LBBB. What do you do now?

_____

_____

c Investigations show normal electrolytes, CXR, and serial cardiac enzymes. Short salvoes of VT are noted during cardiac monitoring. What are the therapeutic options?

_____

_____

Q6 **These drugs are used in secondary prevention following myocardial infarction.**

Aspirin   Fibrate

Beta blockers   ACE inhibitors

Verapamil   Nitrates

Diltiazem   Hydralazine

Statin   Anticoagulants

Which are appropriate for the following patients?

a 45-year-old male smoker, inferior MI, admission cholesterol 6.4, no complications

b 63-year-old diabetic woman, obese, non-smoker, anterior MI, transient heart failure. Admission cholesterol not measured

c 72-year-old man, anterior MI, previous hypertension. No complications. Cholesterol status unknown.

d 66-year-old man, previous CABG, chronic asthma, non-Q wave MI, transient heart failure. Intolerant of aspirin. Cholesterol 6.8.

e 78-year-old woman, inferior MI, heart failure, cholesterol 8.2, remains in AF. Previous hypertension, intolerant of ACEI.

Q7 **In the UK at present, the hospital mortality of patients with heart failure is 20-25%. Which of the following factors are independently related to an adverse prognosis?**

a	BP on admission of > 180mmHg	
b	Plasma urea > 15 mmol/l	
c	Associated myocardial infarction	
d	Age	
e	Gender	
f	Co-morbidity	
g	$Na^+ < 130$ mmol/l	
h	$K^+ < 3.0$ mmol/l	

Q8 **In aortic stenosis, indicate which of the following statements are true:**

a	The louder the murmur, the more severe the disease	T F
b	Doppler ultrasound can significantly underestimate the gradient	T F
c	Peak incidence in the UK is between ages of 55-65	T F
d	Operation is best decided by serial measurement of LV dimensions on echocardiography	T F
e	Pulse pressure may be normal in significant aortic stenosis	T F

Q9 **In mitral stenosis, which of the following statements are true?**

a	The best available treatment for suitable patients is mitral valvoplasty	T F
b	The longer the murmur, the more severe the lesion	T F
c	Doppler ultrasound can overestimate the gradient	T F
d	A pliant valve is indicated by a soft first heart sound	T F
e	Anticoagulants are not indicated in AF if the heart rate is satisfactorily controlled on digoxin	T F

Q10 A 48-year-old restaurant owner presents with progressive dyspnoea and ankle oedema over the course of a month. He is a non-smoker but has been a Type 2 diabetic for ten years and is currently taking metformin and glibenclamide. Clinically he is in sinus tachycardia with signs of left and right heart failure and a pansystolic murmur (3/6) at the apex, associated with an S3 gallop. His CXR shows gross cardiomegaly and the ECG LBBB.

a What is your immediate management?

_____

_____

b List four possible cardiac diagnoses:

1 _____

2 _____

3 _____

4 _____

c Echocardiography shows a grossly dilated and poorly functioning LV (ejection fraction 22%) with mild to moderate mitral regurgitation. There is akinesia of the anteroapical segments of the LV. Which is the most likely diagnosis now?

_____

_____

d What further investigations are necessary to clarify the diagnosis?

_____

_____

Q11 The following groups of drugs are used in the treatment of hypertension

Diuretics – thiazide or loop

Beta blockers – selective and non-selective

Ca channel blockers – dihydropyridine and non-dihydropyridine

ACEI

Alpha blockers

Angiotensin II blockers

Centrally acting vasodilator

Give first choice of drug in the following situations, and the reason why.

a A 48-year-old asymptomatic man with positive FH

b A 35-year-old woman in the last trimester of pregnancy

c A 62-year-old woman with insulin dependent diabetes

d A 78-year-old woman with systolic hypertension

e A 68-year-old woman with bronchitis and paroxysmal AF

Q12 A 74-year-old man is brought in after having blacked out in the street. He has chronic bronchitis and takes tablets for high blood pressure. List four possible causes for the incident and the reason for and against your choice

1 _____

2 _____

3 _____

4 _____

Q13 A 56-year-old woman with paroxysmal AF is admitted with a further episode lasting 12 hours. She is currently taking sotalol 80mg bd. She feels uncomfortable and slightly breathless, but has had no chest pain. The pulse is 110 irregular, the BP 120/80 and the CXR is normal. Which of the following are appropriate treatment strategies?

a Intravenous digoxin

b Immediate DC cardioversion

c Intravenous flecainide

d Intravenous amiodarone

e Anticoagulation with warfarin

Q14 In atrial fibrillation, anticoagulants

a Are contra indicated in the presence of hypertension   T   F

b Are indicated in patients with cardiomegaly in CXR   T   F

c Should not be prescribed without an echocardiogram   T   F

d Are contra-indicated over the age of 75   T   F

e Can be discontinued after successful cardioversion   T   F

Q15 **List the five most important actions in the FAST TRACK management of acute myocardial infarction**

1 _____

2 _____

3 _____

4 _____

5 _____

Q16 **In a patient with acute chest pain, which of the following are true?**

a Sudden onset of pain is classical of inferior MI T F

b Pericarditis is unlikely in the absence of a pericardial rub T F

c Cardiac rupture is more common after thrombolysis T F

d Aortic dissection can be complicated by an inferior MI T F

e Transthoracic echo is the best way of diagnosing aortic dissection in the emergency situation T F

Q17 **In acute myocardial infarction, which of the following statements are true?**

a In inferior MI, right ventricular infarction carries a worse prognosis T F

b Ventricular septal rupture presents with acute pulmonary oedema T F

c Transient heart failure is less important in long term prognosis han early ventricular fibrillation T F

d Cardiogenic shock in anterior myocardial infarction is due to myocardial hibernation T F

e Hypotension associated with RV infarction is best treated with intravenous colloid T F

f ST-depression infarct carries a worse prognosis than ST-elevation infarct T F

Q18 **A patient with an inferior MI is successfully thrombolysed with streptokinase with resolution of ST elevation. Later that night you are called because of further chest pain and ECG elevation in the same leads. What is your management plan?**

_____

_____

_____

_____

Q19 **Which of the following statements about cardiac pacemakers is true?**

a Thrombo-embolism is common in complete heart block and should be prevented by prophylactic anti-coagulants   **T   F**

b Sick sinus syndrome is best treated by an AAIR pacemaker   **T   F**

c Pacemaker syndrome is due to retrograde conduction of the pacemaker impulse from the ventricle to the atrium in DDD pacemakers   **T   F**

d Bifascicular block is an indication for a prophylactic pacemaker even in asymptomatic subjects   **T   F**

e Heart block following anterior myocardial infarction rarely requires a permanent pacemaker   **T   F**

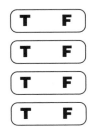

GROUP 11: Respiratory

Q1 **Q1 ABG results pH 7.2, PaO_2 8.5, $PaCO_2$ 13.6, HCO_3 45, (FiO_2 40%)**
Are the following are true or false?

a	Acute respiratory failure	T F
b	A combined respiratory and metabolic acidosis	T F
c	Urgent need for intubation	T F
d	Consistent with acute oxygen toxicity in COPD	T F

Q2 **An anxious asthmatic man of 20 comes to A&E very breathless.**
His PEF is 75l/min. Oximeter reading on air is 86%.
Are the following true or false?

a	No more than 28% O_2 should be used	T F
b	High dose nebulised salbutamol in oxygen should be given	T F
c	IV aminophylline is first line of treatment	T F
d	His anxiety should be treated with sedation	T F

Q3 **A man with a flail chest after an RTA becomes agitated and confused**
with a respiratory rate of six breaths per minute

a	The $PaCO_2$ will be raised	T F
b	Doxapram IV is indicated	T F
c	Arterial blood gases are indicated	T F
d	Excessive analgesia is the likely cause	T F
e	Oxygen is the treatment of choice	T F

Q4 **A 65-year-old man has a major haemoptysis > 250ml/24 hrs**

a	Malignancy is almost certainly the cause	T F
b	Urgent bronchoscopy is necessary	T F
c	An underlying coagulopathy is likely	T F
d	Bronchial artery embolisation may be indicated	T F

Q5 A 35-year-old man complains of intermittent left submammary pain and dizziness for one month

a	Myocardial infarction is unlikely	T	F
b	Pneumothorax is a possible cause	T	F
c	An urgent V/Q scan is indicated	T	F
d	A more detailed history is necessary	T	F

Q6 A 70-year-old smoker complains of increasing wheeze which has not responded to inhalers given for asthma by his GP. Are the following true or false?

a	His eye drops may be the cause	T	F
b	He has developed a pneumothorax	T	F
c	He needs more intensive treatment for asthma	T	F
d	A flow volume loop may be helpful	T	F
e	Bronchoscopy is the next appropriate investigation	T	F

Q7 A 65-year-old smoker complains of increasing breathlessness and hypersomnolence. His wife is concerned by his colour. Are the following true or false?

a	The most likely cause is anaemia	T	F
b	Measurement of spirometric lung volumes may be necessary	T	F
c	As required oxygen could be helpful	T	F
d	Obstructive sleep apnoea is a possibility	T	F

Q8 The following are options for pain control in patients with lung cancer

a Paracetamol

b Slow release morphine tablet

c Dihydrocodeine

d Non-steroidal anti-inflammatory drug

e Fentanyl patches

f Amitryptiline

g Local radiotherapy

h Dexamethasone

i Patient controlled analgesia with diamorphine infusion

For each patient select the most appropriate option(s) for pain relief. Each option can be used once, more than once, or not at all.

a A 65-year-old male with pain in the right thigh due to metastatic deposit in the femur.

_____

_____

b A 70-year-old lady with small cell carcinoma, developed pain in the lower thoracic region in the back with radiation to the front, six months following chemotherapy. Bone scan showed a lytic lesion in D10

_____

_____

c A 56-year-old male developed severe headache 12 months after surgical resection of squamous cell cancer in the left lower lobe. CT scan of the head showed two opacities in the right and one in the left cerebrum

_____

_____

Q9 **A 65-year-old woman presented to A&E with a large pleural effusion. The tuberculosis test is Grade II positive. Are the following true or false?**

a This tuberculosis result indicates TB is the cause   T   F

b No more than 500mls should be drained immediately because of the danger of re-expansion pulmonary oedema   T   F

c Cytology of the pleural fluid is more likely than a blind pleural biopsy to give the result in malignancy   T   F

d Thoracoscopy is often diagnostic when simple aspiration and biopsy prove negative   T   F

Q10 **A 55-year-old with chronic renal failure attends the hospital for haemodialysis. He developed fever and a non-productive cough. The CXR shows bilateral pleural effusions, a perihilar shadowing and infiltration in the right upper lobe. Are the following true or false?**

a Initial treatment with amoxicillin and erythromycin is indicated   T   F

b The tubercular test is a reliable test for TB in these circumstances   T   F

c Bronchoscopy and lavage may be helpful if there is no response to initial antibiotic therapy   T   F

d The sputum is +ve for AFB. Standard triple therapy should be started   T   F

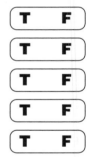

Q11 **A young man was admitted with a ten day history of fever and a productive cough. He has failed to respond to amoxycillin prescribed one week previously. He smokes heavily and admits to drinking approximately 25 units of alcohol a week. The CXR showed right upper lobe consolidation with cavitation. Are the following true or false?**

a Amoxicillin and erythromycin is inadequate treatment   T   F

b TB is a likely cause   T   F

c *Staph aureus* was grown from his sputum. Is this likely to be the causative organism?   T   F

d An HIV test is indicated   T   F

Q12 **A 50-year-old smoker attends A&E with sudden onset breathlessness. The X-ray shows a large right-sided pneumothorax. He reports that he had a collapsed lung on the same side two years previously. The A&E registrar suggests you perform chest aspiration rather than place an intercostal drain. Indicate which statements are true and which are false**

a Aspiration only indicated in shallow pneumothoraces when underlying lung disease unlikely   T   F

b This patient should have a surgical pleurodesis   T   F

c If successfully aspirated, this patient can safely be discharged   T   F

d Failure of lung to re expand with tube drainage indicates urgent need for surgery   T   F

e Chest tube may be safely removed when bubbling has stopped   T   F

Q13 **A 32-year-old female presents with a swollen leg and suspected pulmonary embolism**

a What immediate investigations would be conducted in the A&E department?

_____

_____

b What additional information would you seek from the patient assuming the diagnosis is confirmed?

_____

_____

_____

Q14 **A 55-year-old asthmatic presents with a ten day history of increased wheeze and sudden deterioration on day of arrival in A&E.**
He is agitated and ABG on air are pH 7.35, pO$_2$ 6.8, pCO$_2$ 7.4.
Are the following true or false?

a These ABG results indicate need for intubation   T   F

b Aminophylline indicated if no response to nebulised salbutamol and ipratropium   T   F

c Non-invasive ventilation should be tried if available prior to intubation and IPPV   T   F

d Cautious sedation appropriate to manage his agitation   T   F

e IV magnesium is of potential benefit in acute asthma   T   F

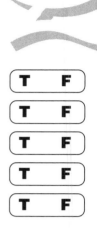

GROUP 12: ITU

Q1 The following are causes of shock

a	Pulmonary embolism	T F
b	Pericarditis	T F
c	Urinary tract infection	T F
d	Wasp sting	T F
e	*Giardia intestinalis* infection	T F

Q2 The following are features of hypovolaemic shock

a	Cold pale skin	T F
b	Tachycardia	T F
c	Normal blood pressure	T F
d	Metabolic alkalosis	T F
e	Oliguria	T F

Q3 Concerning acute respiratory distress syndrome (ARDS)

a	The outcome depends on the underlying cause	T F
b	The outcome depends on the severity of the lung injury	T F
c	The main aim of therapy is to improve tissue oxygenation	T F
d	Many patients respond to immediate antibiotic therapy	T F
e	Pneumothorax is a recognised complication	T F

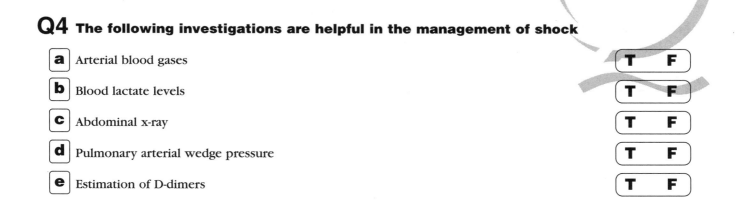

Q4 The following investigations are helpful in the management of shock

a	Arterial blood gases	**T**	**F**
b	Blood lactate levels	**T**	**F**
c	Abdominal x-ray	**T**	**F**
d	Pulmonary arterial wedge pressure	**T**	**F**
e	Estimation of D-dimers	**T**	**F**

Q5 Discuss the differences between acute septicaemic, haemorrhagic and cardiogenic shock

_____

_____

_____

_____

_____

_____

Q6 Discuss the clinical presentation of ARDS and the main approaches to management

_____

_____

_____

_____

_____

_____

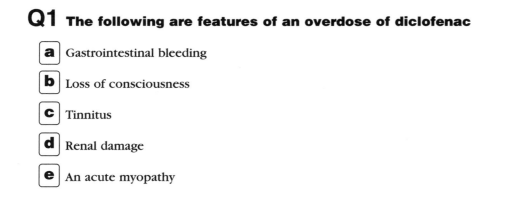

GROUP 13: Poisoning

Q1 The following are features of an overdose of diclofenac

a Gastrointestinal bleeding   T   F

b Loss of consciousness   T   F

c Tinnitus   T   F

d Renal damage   T   F

e An acute myopathy   T   F

Q2 The following substances are poorly absorbed by activated charcoal

a Carbamazepine   T   F

b Ethylene glycol   T   F

c Lithium   T   F

d Phenytoin   T   F

e Iron   T   F

Q3 Features of neuroleptic malignant syndrome include

a Muscular atony   T   F

b Autonomic dysfunction   T   F

c A raised creatine phosphokinase   T   F

d Hyperthermia   T   F

e Bradycardia   T   F

Q4 A 16-year-old girl is admitted following an overdose of a single drug. After initial assessment you do her blood gases which show:
$PaO_2 = 13.5kPa$, $PaCO_2 = 2.8kPa$, $[H+] = 29$ nmoles/l

a What do these blood gases indicate?

_____

_____

_____

b What drug has she taken?

_____

_____

_____

c How would you assess her future suicidal risk state?

_____

_____

_____

_____

Q5 How would you manage a patient with an acute overdose of digoxin taken one hour prior to being seen in A&E?

_____

_____

_____

_____

Q6 Self poisoning is common. True or false?

T   F

Q7 Name the three most common drugs used in overdoses in the UK

1 _____

2 _____

3 _____

Q8 **Name two other drugs available OTC that are associated with self-poisoning**

1 _____

2 _____

Q9 **What is the overall mortality following self-poisoning?**

<1%   [   ]

1-5%   [   ]

>5%   [   ]

Q10 **What six principles underpin the management of self-poisoning?**

1 _____

2 _____

3 _____

4 _____

5 _____

6 _____

Q11 **Regarding overdose**

a It is common for overdose to be complicated by more than one drug ingestion. True or false?   [**T   F**]

b Name the second commonest drug

_____

Q12 **You should not induce emesis/gastric lavage after the following overdose**

a Paraquat   [**T   F**]

b Petrol   [**T   F**]

c Corrosive   [**T   F**]

d Theophylline   [**T   F**]

Q13 **What is the time frame for gastric lavage?**

a < 4 hours

b 4-12 hours

c >12 hours

Q14 **What can you do to enhance drug elimination if gastric lavage is contra-indicated?**

_____

_____

_____

Q15 **Emesis can be used to reduce absorption in the unconscious patient. True or false?**

T   F

Q16 **Name three drugs for which active charcoal works to reduce absorption**

1 _____

2 _____

3 _____

Q17 **You need to administer antibiotics for a community-acquired chest infection to a patient who has overdosed on tricyclic anti-depressants. What antibiotics class would you avoid and why?**

_____

_____

_____

_____

Q18 **Does active elimination have a role in overdoses and with what drugs?**

_____

_____

_____

_____

Q19 **Name three antidotes for drugs of overdose and give examples of use**

1 _____

2 _____

3 _____

Q20 **Is there anything special about a suspected ecstasy overdose?**

_____

_____

_____

Q21 **A young woman is brought into A&E unconscious**

a Describe how you would assess her in A&E

_____

_____

_____

_____

b Intravenous access is obtained and fluids started based on the observation above.

A urinary catheter is also be inserted and the patient is attached to an ECG monitor.
Bloods should be taken for what?

_____

_____

c What drugs should you request for screening?

_____

_____

d You conduct an exam and find nil of note. What immediate further care would you order to ensure the safety of the patient?

_____

_____

e The drug screen returned two hours later showing high levels of tricyclic anti-depressants. What significance does that information add to her ongoing management?

_____

_____

_____

_____

Q22 **You are required to look after two young patients with paracetamol overdose, the first ingested the drug no more than two hours before arriving in A&E (P1) and the second ingested the drug at least 30 hours ago (P2). Compare and contrast their management as requested below.**

a What are the likely differences in symptoms expressed by these two patients?

_____

_____

b What are the differences in emergency treatment?

_____

_____

c Patient two (P2) is known to be HIV+ and is on anti TB therapy. Does this information affect your decision concerning NAC and why?

_____

_____

d With whom would you discuss what to do with patient two: the poisons centre or the liver unit?

_____

e Which of the following blood tests are crucial to the ongoing monitoring of both patients and why?

FBC

U&E/Creat

INR (prothrombin time)

Paracetamol level

LFTs

Q23 What is the best chance of recovery of someone in FHF?

_____

_____

_____

_____

GROUP 14: Endocrinology

Q1 **The following patients are likely to have a reduced radioactive iodine uptake when scanned**

a A patient with untreated Graves disease   T   F

b A patient with untreated hypothyroidism   T   F

c A patient on propylthoiuracil   T   F

d A patient within 24 hours of the onset of neck pain who has viral (de Quervains) thyroiditis and who is clinically and biochemically thyrotoxic   T   F

e The patient in (d), but a month later when he is clinically and biochemically hypothyroid   T   F

f In a patient who is on maintanence amiodarone   T   F

g In a patient who discontinued amiodarone a month ago   T   F

Q2 **A patient presents with severe breathlessness to A&E. On direct questioning he says he has been losing weight for four months. Examination reveals a tachycardia at 170 bpm and he is pyrexial 41ºC. He has a raised JVP and bilateral basal crackles. He also has dullness to percussion, increased vocal resonance and bronchial breathing at the right base, consistent with a right lower lobar pneumonia. Thyroid function tests are sent together with the other usual blood tests for a patient with pneumonia and heart failure, and reveal thyrotoxicosis**

a What is the diagnosis?

_____

_____

_____

_____

b How will the discovery of the thyrotoxicosis alter your management?

_____

_____

_____

_____

c Where should this patient be managed?

_____

_____

_____

_____

d What treatment is required?

_____

_____

_____

_____

Q3 A patient with known Addison's disease presents to A&E having lost
his hydrocortisone and fludrocortisone tablets. He says he has not had
any for three days. On examination he has a tachycardia of 120bpm,
and is hypotensive (90/60) with a postural drop (70/30).
Investigations confirm hyperkalaemia and hyponatraemia.
What emergency treatment does he need?

_____

_____

_____

_____

Q4 A 45-year-old lady has an incidentally discovered calcium of 2.85 mmol/l
and a phosphate of 0.5 mmol/l. The PTH is 2.8 (normal range 1.1-6.8).
What is the most likely diagnosis?

_____

_____

_____

_____

Q5 A patient with primary hyperparathyroidism is found at surgery to have a solitary parathyroid adenoma, which is excised. Postoperatively, her calcium falls from 2.95 to 1.95. How should this patient be monitored and what treatment does she need?

_____

_____

_____

_____

Q6 A patient wth primary hyperparathyroidism is found at surgery to have four gland hyperplasia. The surgeon therefore removes all four parathyroid glands. Postoperatively, her calcium falls from 2.95 to 1.95 mmol/l.

a What diagnosis must be considered?

_____

_____

b How should this patient be monitored and what treatment does she need ?

_____

_____

c What is your target calcium?

_____

Q7 The following are at increased risk of hypertension due to phaeochromocytoma

a An individual with a previously removed papillary thyroid carcinoma   **T**   **F**

b An individual with a previously removed medullary thyroid carcinoma   **T**   **F**

c An individual whose mother has previously had a papillary thyroid carcinoma   **T**   **F**

d An indvidual whose mother has previoulsy had a medullary thyroid carcinoma   **T**   **F**

e An individual with Von-Recklinghausan's disease (neurofibromatosis)   **T**   **F**

f An individual with Von-Hippel Lindau disease   **T**   **F**

g An individual with renal artery stenosis   **T**   **F**

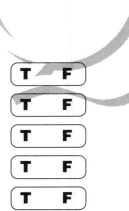

Q8 Are the following statements true or false?

a Addison's disease is associated with hyperpigmentation T F

b Cushing's disease is associated with hyperpigmentation T F

c Postural hypotension is more severe in Sheehan's syndrome than in Addison's disease T F

d Pituitary infarction often occurs in males who develop hypovolaemic shock T F

e Pituitary infarction only occurs in females who are pregnant and who also develop hypovolaemic shock T F

Q9 You are called urgently to the psychiatric wing of your hospital to see a 41-year-old long term manic depressive who has just had an epileptic fit. He has been on maintenance lithium carbonate for several months, and the most recent lithium level is in the middle of the therapeutic range. Urgent biochemistry reveals: Na 117, K 4.6, U 5.0, Cr 100, Glucose 4.9 mmol/l. The measured plasma osmolality is 256 and a urine dipstick reveals a specific gravity of 1.001. What is the likely diagnosis?

_____

_____

_____

_____

Q10 Are the following statements true or false?

a Patients with type 1 diabetes may be unconscious due to a low pH T F

b Patients with type 2 diabetes may be unconscious due to a high plasma osmolality T F

c The commonest cause of a patient known to have diabetes arriving unconscious in casualty is hypoglycaemia T F

d Metformin overdoses can cause severe hypoglycaemia T F

e A patient with stable type 1 diabetes on 40 units of insulin daily can safely be advised to discontinue his insulin for 24 hours if he develops vomiting, because if he cannot keep any food down he is at serious risk of hypoglycaemic coma T F

f A patient with stable type 2 diabetes on 40 units of insulin daily can safely be advised to discontinue his insulin for 24 hours for any reason T F

g IM glucagon is effective treatment for hypoglycaemia by stimulating breakdown of stored hepatic glycogen T F

h During pregnancy, patients usually need to increase their dose of insulin regularly T F

GROUP 15: Neurology

Q1 **A 19-year-old first-year university student felt unwell last night and woke up with a headache, muscular aches, nausea and vomiting. On arrival in A&E at 11am she was drowsy and disoriented. On examination, she had a temperature of 38.5°C, a pulse of 120/min, blood pressure 100/60 and a purpuric rash**

a What is your clinical diagnosis?

b How would you manage her immediately?

c What tests would you do?

d What other factors would you address?

Q2 **The following are causes of a VIth nerve palsy**

a	Diabetes mellitus	T F
b	Acoustic neuroma	T F
c	Motor neurone disease	T F
d	Raised intracranial pressure	T F
e	Head injury	T F

Q3 **A 70-year-old man presents with difficulty in walking. This was partly due to pain in his buttocks on walking, but he also complained of stiffness in the legs. On further questioning he admitted to difficulty in doing up his shirt buttons. He smoked 30 cigarettes a per day but considered himself fit. On examination he had a mild spastic quadriparesis but the ankle jerks were absent. Peripheral pulses were palpable and his feet were warm**

a What is the diagnosis?

b What investigations would you do?

c How would you treat?

Q4 **Name the three most common causes of avoidable blindness world-wide. The term 'avoidable' blindness describes diseases either preventable or reversible by easily available interventions**

1 _____

2 _____

3 _____

Q5 **A 45-year-old lady was admitted with extreme weakness of her legs. On examination she had gross wasting of her proximal muscles of her legs. In addition, she had decreased sensation to pin prick and to light touch distally and absent ankle jerks. Her GP had already performed some routine blood tests: Hb 12.1g/dl, MCV 102fl, Bilirubin 20 µmol/l, Albumin 39 g/l, ALT 150 IU/l, ALP 180 IU/l**

a What are the diagnoses?

_____

_____

b Explain the findings

_____

_____

_____

_____

Q6 **A 30-year-old man is brought to A&E having had a fit. He is now well and tells you that ten years ago he had a similar episode and was seen by a neurologist. He was told the diagnosis was epilepsy and was prescribed phenytoin which he took for one year. His main concern now is whether he can drive his car as he is a sales rep.**
What advice would you give him?

_____

_____

_____

_____

_____

_____

_____

_____

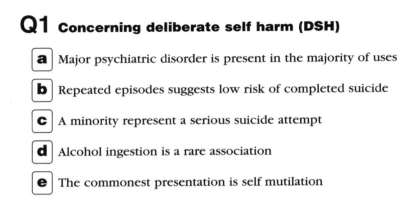

GROUP 16: Psychiatry

Q1 Concerning deliberate self harm (DSH)

a Major psychiatric disorder is present in the majority of uses   T   F

b Repeated episodes suggests low risk of completed suicide   T   F

c A minority represent a serious suicide attempt   T   F

d Alcohol ingestion is a rare association   T   F

e The commonest presentation is self mutilation   T   F

Q2 In the assesment of DSH the following are associated with increased suicide risk

a Major depressive illness   T   F

b Psychotic symptoms   T   F

c Middle age   T   F

d Chronic painful illness   T   F

e Being married   T   F

Q3 You are called to see a 57-year-old man, an inpatient for two weeks with complications of lung cancer. The nurses describe variations in his behaviour and are concerned because he has been refusing care, accusing them of trying to harm him

a What may be causing his persecuting ideas and strange behaviour?

_____

_____

_____

_____

b You find evidence of disorientation and impaired conciousness. Does this suggest a particular diagnosis and what other features may be present?

_____

_____

_____

c How would you clarify the diagnosis?

_____

_____

_____

_____

d How would you manage this patient?

_____

_____

_____

_____

Q4 A patient on the ward tells you she feels depressed. What features of the mental state examination would suggest a major depressive illness and when would an urgent psychiatric assessment be needed?

_____

_____

_____

_____

Q5 Symptoms of acute withdrawal from heroin (diamorphine)

a Often include convulsions · T · F

b Are reversed by administering naloxone · T · F

c Last longer than the symptoms which follow acute withdrawal from methadone · T · F

d Are mainly psychological · T · F

e If untreated are life threatening · T · F

Q6 A 24-year-old man is brought to A&E by his family. He has developed rigidity in his arms and legs. He complains of stiffness in his facial muscles and tongue causing him to dribble profusely. You discover he has been taking haloperidol 15mg daily for the past week.

a What is the likely problem?

_____

_____

_____

_____

b How would you manage this man?

_____

_____

_____

_____

c On examination you find he is pyrexial. His observations are unstable with fluctuating blood pressure and pulse. He has clouded consciousness. With particular reference to his current medication what other diagnosis would you consider and would any investigation support this?

_____

_____

_____

_____

d What further management is required?

_____

_____

_____

_____

GROUP 17: Dermatology

Q1 **Write short notes on toxic epidermal necrolysis (TEN)**

_____
_____
_____
_____
_____
_____
_____

Q2 **What is eczema herpeticum, and how is it treated?**

_____
_____
_____
_____

Q3 **What skin conditions may also involve mucosal surfaces?**

_____
_____
_____
_____

Q4 **In a patient with a swollen red leg, which specific areas of skin should also be examined?**

_____
_____
_____
_____

Q5 **What is your differential diagnosis of a swollen hot red leg?**

_____
_____
_____

Q6 **What investigations would you do for suspected cellulitis?**

Q7 **You admit the patient with cellulitis for IV antibiotics (benzyl penicillin and flucloxacillin) and mark the limit of the cellulitis with a marker pen. 24 hours later the cellulitis has progressed 5cm and areas of black necrosis appear. The patient remains unwell. So far your investigations have shown a neutrophilia, an ESR of 95 and diabetes. What must you consider?**

Q8 **A 16-year-old unmarried Asian girl presents to an inner city A&E with her mother. She has painful red lumps on her skin and arthralgia. Walking has become painful. She is otherwise well with no relevant PMH.**

a What other specific questions would you ask her?

b On examination you feel deep very tender red lumps on the shins and make a clinical diagnosis of erythema nodosum. How would you investigate her?

c No cause is found. How would you treat her?

_____

_____

_____

_____

Q9 **A 22-year-old woman presents in A&E with a six-hour history of a florid raised red rash all over the body. It is very itchy and distressing and has caused swelling around her eyes and her right hand.**

a What questions would you ask her?

_____

_____

_____

_____

_____

b Your above thorough history reveals nothing. However she did suffer with atopic eczema as a child and gets mild hayfever. She has had a similar rash in a milder form on and off for about three weeks. Examining her you find red, raised weals and periorbital swelling. What is your diagnosis and the likely cause?

_____

_____

_____

c How would you manage this patient?

_____

_____

_____

_____

d Should you check her C1 esterase inhibitor level?

_____

Q10 A 50-year-old farmer attends A&E with a widespread non-itchy blistering eruption and painful mouth ulceration which has stopped him from eating. PMH and DH are nil. On examination he has multiple, well-circumscribed erythematous lesions some of which are blistering. He has a few blistering lesions on the palms and soles and marked erosions of the tongue, lower lip and palate

a What is the likely diagnosis?

_____

_____

_____

_____

b What is your differential diagnosis of the triad 'rash, blisters, mucosal erosion'?

_____

_____

_____

_____

c In the above patient, what is the differential diagnosis of a blistering eruption if there are no oral lesions?

_____

_____

_____

_____

d The farmer has a plaster on his right index finger. Underneath is a boil which he has had for two to three weeks. Why might he have erythema multiforme (EM)?

_____

_____

_____

_____

e What are the other causes of EM?

_____

_____

_____

f How would you manage his EM?

_____

_____

_____

Q11 **A 63-year-old gentleman presents in A&E unwell, shivering and red all over. He has suffered with chronic plaque psoriasis for 40 years and has been managed on topical therapy only. He smells of alcohol and admits to being a heavy drinker. He was recently diagnosed with a meningioma and had been commenced on carbamazepine three weeks previously for the control of fits. Examination reveals erythroderma and multiple tiny pustules over the trunk. He has a pyrexia of 39.5°C and is clinically dehydrated. He is alert with no neurological signs.**

a What are the first things you would do?

_____

_____

_____

_____

b What diagnoses are likely?

_____

_____

_____

_____

c What tests would help distinguish these?

_____

_____

_____

_____

d What are the complications of erythroderma?

_____

_____

_____

_____

e Investigations suggest ACHS. If cabamazepine is stopped, what other antiepileptic can be used in this man?

_____

_____

Q12 A 19-year-old white man presents with a six-week history of an itchy skin which has been 'driving him mad' especially at night-time and he can't sleep. He is fed up with his GP who said he had scabies and has treated him four times with malathion without benefit. PMH/SH Nil. He had bad asthma as a child. On examination he had multiple small red papules on trunk, around nipples, wrists, axillae and on the penis. These were accompanied by marked excoriations. No burrows were seen. A few lesions were seen on the soles of the feet.

a At this stage what diagnoses should be considered?

_____

_____

_____

_____

b What points in history should be looked at?

_____

_____

_____

_____

c The diagnosis of scabies was made on clinical grounds. Burrows are not always present but the distribution of non-specific papules (occasionally vesicles) is highly suggestive. Sites commonly involved are axillae nipples, penis, wrists, palms, soles and web spaces. The face/head is spared in adults. Scabies can be confirmed by skin scraping and microscopy. He lived with his girlfriend (who was unaffected) and had recently visited a prostitute who may have been the source of infection. Why might he not have responded to treatment?

_____

_____

_____

_____

Q13 A 25-year-old female presents with a two-day history of a widespread rash all over the body. It is mildly itchy but she is otherwise well

a What would you ask?

_____

_____

_____

_____

b On examination she has multiple non-specific red macules and small papules on the trunk and limbs and a few on the face. There is no mucosal involvement or lymphodenopathy. Two weeks before she had had headaches and a sore throat and was treated with amoxicillin by her GP. What diagnoses are possible?

_____

_____

_____

_____

c What investigations would you perform to elucidate the diagnosis?

_____

_____

_____

_____

GROUP 1: Infectious diseases

A1

 False

Patients with infections due to *S.typhi* usually have a low normal or low peripheral white cell count with decreased polymorphs and slightly low platelet count. This is unusual as with most bacterial infections the peripheral white cell count classically increases

b **False**

Cefuroxime is inappropriate therapy for typhoid. Ciprofloxacin is the treatment of choice for adults

c **True**

d **False**

Most types of salmonella have an animal reservoir. *S. typhi* is the exception – humans are the reservoir

e **True**

A2

a **False**

If a lumbar puncture is done in a patient with raised intracranial pressure there is a danger that the patient might 'cone'. Prior to lumbar puncture the patient should be examined for papilloedema and focal neurological signs to look for raised intracranial pressure. A CT scan should also be done in any unconscious patient

b **True**

Septicaemia due to *N. meningitidis* is frequently rapidly fulminant and may not be recognised in the early stages

c **False**

There is a vaccine currently available for contacts of *N. meningitidis* types A, C, V and W135 but not against type B which is the commonest serotype in the UK

d **False**

Rifampicin prophylaxis should only be given to close contacts of patients with *N. meningitidis*. Staff who have specialed/resuscitated the patient during the first 24-48 hours after admission require prophylaxis

e **True**

Rifampicin causes many secretions to be coloured e.g. tears and urine. It also decreases the efficacy of the oral contraceptive pill and any females prescribed rifampicin should be warned of this and advised to take additional contraceptive precautions

Other comments

Management for meningococcal meningitis/septicaemia is an emergency.

Provide supportive therapy. Take blood and throat cultures and then start antibiotics IMMEDIATELY. Give intravenous benzylpenicillin initially 2.4g four hourly or IV cefotaxime 2g six hourly or IV ceftriaxone 2g/day for presumed meningococcal meningitis/septicaemia. If it is thought that a patient could have bacterial meningitis caused by *S. pneumoniae* you should commence treatment on cefotaxime or ceftriaxone and not an IV benzylpenicillin since 5-10% of *S. pneumoniae* in the U.K. have decreased susceptibility to penicillin. If *Haemophilus influenzae* is suspected as a possible cause (rare in children over the age of 5 years and also now uncommon in the U.K. due to vaccination) cefotaxime or ceftriaxone should also be given. If the other causes of septicaemia cannot be excluded broader spectrum antimicrobial therapy may be required

A3

a Pseudomembranous colitis is caused by toxin producing strains of *Clostridium difficile*. The diagnosis is initially a clinical one. It usually occurs in patients who have recently received/are receiving broad spectrum antimicrobial therapy. Sigmoidoscopy may show an erythematous ulcerated mucosa covered by a membrane-like material but a normal sigmoidoscopy does not exclude infection. A stool should be sent to the microbiology department specifically requesting *C. difficile* culture and toxin in addition to standard microscopy, culture and sensitivity. To make the diagnosis of pseudomembranous colitis a stool should be *C. difficile* toxin positive since some normal people will carry *C. difficile* in their stool. NB Most laboratories will not routinely look for *C. difficile* in the stool so it must be specifically requested

b Administration of broad spectrum antibiotics – especially those which are relatively poorly absorbed and so are present in large amounts in the gastrointestinal tract will cause much of the normal intestinal flora to be removed and so make the GI tract more susceptible to colonisation with *C. difficile*. Virtually all antibiotics have been implicated in causing pseudomembranous colitis. Clindamycin was probably the most heavily implicated in the 1970s – 1980s and this led to a great reduction in its use. Ceftazidine and broad spectrum penicillins are also fairly commonly implicated.

c Isolate the patient in a side-room with (if possible) excretion - secretion precautions. Supportive therapy – as required. Stop any antibiotics the patient is on (if at all possible). Give oral metronidazole 400mg x three per day for seven to ten days or oral vancomycin 125-250 mg x four per day for ten days.

A4

a **False**

Chickenpox in children (excluding neonates) has much lower complications than in adults: pneumonia is much commoner in adults and has a significant morbidity especially in smokers and in pregnancy. The immunosuppressed are also likely to have severe disseminated disease due to VZV. Early treatment with aciclovir should always be given to the immunosuppressed if they develop an infection due to VZV and should be considered in all adults

b **True**

c **False**

A patient with shingles may give chickenpox to a susceptible host. Virus is disseminated from freshly formed vesicles

d **True**

e **True**

To be at its most effective aciclovir should be given as early as possible and certainly within the first 72 hours of lesions developing

f **False**

A streptococcus (*S. pyogenes*) and *S. aureus* are the commonest secondary bacterial infection in shingles

A5

a **False**

A recent multicentre European study found about 70 per cent of bacteraemia to be nosocomial

b **True**

Intravenous catheters are the commonest single cause of nosocomial bacteraemias and account for approximately a third of them. Most of the bacteraemias are from central lines and not from peripheral intravenous catheters

c **False**

Intubation and ventilation are major predisposing factors

d **True**

Litigation due to nosocomial infections is increasing significantly

e **False**

Urinary tract infections are the commonest nosocomial infection and respiratory tract infections are the third most common cause. However, respiratory tract infections have the highest morbidity and mortality

f True

A6

a The term means pyrexia of unknown origin which classically has been of at least three weeks in duration

b You need to obtain a full travel history including exactly where the patient has been eg in town/country and what sort of accommodation they stayed in. Did the patient have the relevant vaccination before she went away? Did she take malaria prophylaxis? Did she sleep under mosquito nets and wear long sleeved shirts and cover her legs? Was there contact with sick animals/people, and if so was the cause of their illness known? What did the patient do while abroad – occupation, water exposure, any risk behaviour etc? Did the patient eat any suspect food or drink dirty water?

c Start with cheap and relatively non-invasive tests. Perform FBC and ESR/CRP, urea and electrolytes, liver function tests. Send urine for microscopy, culture and sensitivity, stools for ova, cysts and parasites and culture and blood cultures. Store serum for future serological tests (if required) and take a repeat serum two weeks later. Perform thick and thin blood films for malaria. Perform other tests as indicated from your history/examination and depending on initial results

d The patient should be admitted to a side-room for isolation until an infection such as S. typhi has been ruled out.

NB In recently returned travellers malaria, typhoid, bacterial gastroenteritis and amoebiasis are important causes of fever. Tuberculosis should also be considered. However, patients may also have fever due to illnesses acquired in the UK eg colds and influenza

GROUP 2: STDs

A1

a **False**

Infections due to *Mycobacterium tuberculosis* can develop early in the course of infection while the patient is only mildly immunosuppressed

b **True**

Most cases of tuberculosis in HIV positive individuals probably represent reactivation of dormant bacilli. However, as the prevalence if both HIV and TB goes up in a community, new infections occur or re-infections will increasingly occur

c **True**

The pattern of disease differs according to the patients' degree of immunosuppression. In patients with relatively well preserved CD4 counts the presentation of respiratory disease due to *Mycobacterium tuberculosis* will be similar to that seen in HIV negative individuals. In more advanced HIV disease atypical presentations are common: patients tend to have less cavitation on CXR, have more lower lobe involvement and more extrapulmonary disease

d **True**

Rifamycin derivatives interact with the protease class of anti-retrovirals resulting in an increase in rifamycin toxicity and reduced protease efficiency. Treatment of these patients requires input from both specialists in HIV and respiratory medicine

e **False**

Mycobacterium avium-intracellulare complex tends to cause infections only in the severely immunosuppressed with very low CD4 counts around 50/mm³. It is an organism of lower pathogenicity than *Mycobacterium tuberculosis*

A2

a **False**

Pneumonia due to *Pneumocystis carinii* frequently has an insidious onset

b **True**

c **True**

The exact CD4 count when anti-PCP prophylaxis starts varies a bit from centre to centre. However, PCP is usually not seen until patients are severely immunosuppressed with a CD4 count of <200/mm³. However, if a patient has already had PCP, secondary life-long prophylaxis should be commenced for them even if their CD4 count is above 200/mm³

d **True**

The abnormalities of B cell function associated with HIV lead to an increased number of infections with encapsulated bacteria. An increased incidence of bacterial sepsis may be seen at early stages of HIV infection. Infections due to *S. pneumoniae* and Salmonella spp are a particular problem in HIV infected indivduals

e **False**

Unlike with *Pneumocystis carinii* pneumonia, respiratory tract infections due to bacteria such as *S. pneumoniae*, *H. influenzae* and *M. catarrhalis* are usually of rapid onset

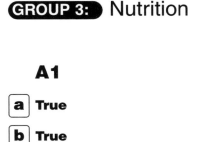

GROUP 3: Nutrition

A1

a True

b True

c False

d True

e False

Hyperglycaemia is common because of the high amount of glucose in the solution. Insulin is usually required. A cholestatic jaundice occurs infrequently but the mechanism is unknown. It has been suggested that it could be due to a fatty liver. Essential fatty acid deficiency was described with the nitrogen/glucose solutions without fat. All modern regimes contain lipids. Pneumothorax occurs as a results of the central catheter which is usually inserted just below the clavicle

A2

a True

b True

c True

d True

e False

The liver is the main storage organ for Vitamin A. Folic acid is added to bread in the UK. This fortification is advocated to reduce neural tubule defects. Vitamin B12 is found in milk. It is not destroyed by boiling. Vitamin K is found in many oily vegetables. Animal sources are a poor source of Vitamin E

A3

Give enough nitrogen in the diet. Hypercatabolic patients require 15g of nitrogen per 24 hours

Monitor weight
Regular serum albumin estimations.
Nitrogen loss can be calculated using the formula:
N_2 loss (g/24hr) = urinary urea (mmols/24hr) x 0.02842 +2

(2 represents non-urinary excretion.)
Urea, as opposed to nitrogen, can be easily measured in urine.

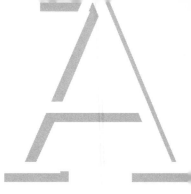

GROUP 4: Gastroenterology

A1

a **False**

Involvement is often patchy but mainly involves the jejunum

b **True**

Oral dapsone also helps the skin lesion

c **True**

Malignant complications include lymphoma, oesophageal cancer and small intestinal cancer

d **False**

The ileum (where B_{12} is absorbed) is often not grossly involved. The B_{12} is often normal. Red cell folate is usually low in untreated disease

e **False**

There is often splenic atrophy with associated Howell-Jolly bodies in red cells

A2

a These features, particularly in a young female, strongly suggest irritable bowel syndrome. Inflammatory bowel disease, particularly Crohn's disease, can also present with pain and alternation of bowel habit but other features, eg weight loss, systemic symptoms, rectal bleeding are often present

b In the young well patient, investigation is often unnecessary. If there is doubt, blood tests to assess inflammatory markers (Hb, WCC, platelets, ESR/CRP, albumen) should be checked. If diarrhoea is a predominant symptom, a rectal biopsy should be performed

c Management of IBS is largely with reassurance. Occasionally anti-spasmodics (eg mebeverine) can be useful. Depression should be actively sought and treated

A3

a The commoner causes of dysphagia include a benign or malignant stricture, motility disorders such as achalasia or oesophageal spasm. Intramuscular disorders such as bulbar palsy and myasthenia gravis and extrinsic pressure such as a lung tumour can cause dysphagia

b A history of heartburn suggests a peptic stricture. Progressive dysphagia with weight loss suggests malignancy. Chest pain, regurgitation and dysphagia for liquids suggest a motility disorder such as achalasia

c A barium swallow is usually the best initial investigation. Endoscopy may be normal in motility disorders. Causes of high dysphagia, e.g. pharyngeal pouch may make endoscopy hazardous

d Treatment depends on patient's age, general health and extent of tumour. Liver biochemistry, CXR, abdominal ultrasound and CT ± endoscopic ultrasound will usually indicate operability and possibility for cure. If inoperable, oesophageal stents can be inserted

e Treatments for achalasia include intrasphincteric injections of botulin toxin, pneumatic balloon dilation of the sphincter, or a surgical cardiomyotomy. Surgical treatment is now most commonly performed laparoscopically and is becoming the treatment of choice

A4

a **False**

Normal stool weight is <250g/24 hours. A complaint of diarrhoea with normal stool weight suggests functional bowel disorder or is commonly proctitis or left sided bowel cancer

b **False**

Campylobacter or shigella can cause bloody diarrhoea but ulcerative colitis is more likely

c **False**

Serum amylase will be normal if pancreatic insufficiency is the cause of diarrhoea

d **True**

Mucosal biopsies should always be taken to exclude microscopic inflammation or rarer conditions such as collapenous colitis. Occasionally colonic disease may be evident only in the right side of the colon, eg Crohn's, pseudomembranous colitis

e **False**

Most causes of infectious diarrhoea are self limiting. Antibiotics are usually only used if the patient is ill or if *C. difficle* is the cause (metronidazole).

A5

a In this age group RIF pain and weight loss strongly suggests Crohn's disease. Other causes of these symptoms would include an appendix mass, though the history is long. In immigrants ileo-caecal TB should be considered. Amoebiasis can cause RIF pain, usually with formation as an amoeboma and should be considered in a traveller returning from the tropics

b Blood tests looking for inflammatory causes – Hb, WCC, ESR, albumin. Ultrasound of the RIF will identify masses and thickened bowel. A small bowel follow through will confirm a diagnosis of Crohn's. Colonoscopy and ileoscopy will provide histological confirmation

c This patient is symptomatic and therefore Crohn's disease requires treatment. Medical options include prednisone 40mg daily reducing over 4 to 6 weeks. 5-ASA drugs (mesalazine) have limited use in ileo-caecal Crohn's but may reduce the risk of relapse, particularly following surgery. Surgery should be considered particularly for limited ileo-caecal disease and for disease associated with stricturing or fistulisation. Other options include elemental feeding (for diffuse disease) and more recently infusion of anti TNF-alpha antibodies

A6

a Most causes of rectal bleeding do not induce haemodynamic compromise. In this scenario the likely cause would be diverticular disease, an ischaemic colon or possibly a vascular abnormality. Cancer and colitis do not usually bleed sufficiently briskly to induce shock

b Resuscitation is the key. A large bore intravenous cannula is inserted and colloid, preferably blood, is infused. Insertion of a CVP line should be considered. Urgent consultation with surgical colleagues is required.

c A history of pain, diarrhoea and weight loss may suggest ischaemia or cancer. Blood tests in the acute stage are often unhelpful. A plain film of the abdomen may show evidence of mucosal oedema/thumb printing. Endoscopic examination of the colon is usually unhelpful in the acute situation but should be scheduled electively if the bleeding stops spontaneously. Angiography may be indicated if bleeding continues and the origin is unclear. Often laparotomy is required if bleeding continues.

A7

a **False**

Although the MCV is reduced in iron deficiency, there are other causes of a low MCV, ie thalassaemia, sideroblastic anaemia. Iron deficiency should be proven with iron studies before proceeding with further investigations

b **False**

The TIBC will be elevated with a low iron and ferritin level

c **True**

Iron deficiency in the absence of menorrhagia must be due to a gastrointestinal disorder. A negative FOB does not exclude a GI cause and further investigation is indicated regardless of the FOB status

d **False**

Folate is absorbed in the jejunum. Terminal ileal resection may lead to B_{12} deficiency

e **True**

In a menstruating female, iron deficiency is common

A8

a **False**

In this age group new onset of symptoms should be investigated before treatment is undertaken

b **False**

The serum amylase is usually normal in chronic pancreatic disease.

c **False**

Serology is not helpful in checking the success or otherwise of *H.pylori* eradication as antibodies persist despite successful treatment. A positive *H.pylori* breath test will indicate current infection

d **True**

In the absence of peptic disease, eradication of *H. pylori* is unlikely to benefit symptoms

e **True**

Recurrence following successful eradication is extremely uncommon

GROUP 5: Liver, biliary and pancreatic disorders

A1

a Ascites may be an exudate, eg abdominal infection (TB) or malignancy or a transudate, eg chronic liver disease with portal hypertension or long term cardiac failure. Protein concentration of the ascitic fluid will differentiate

b Liver biochemistry- to check for liver disease. PT, albumin will assess liver function. A chest X-ray to assess heart size. The ascites should be tapped and a sample sent for protein estimation, white cell count, cytology and amylase. If liver disease is suspected appropriate investigation for viral, metabolic and autoimmune causes of liver disease should be sought

c Ascites due to infection or malignancy are treated according to the underlying cause.

In decompensated liver disease treatment is instituted with bed rest, low salt diet and the aldosterone antagonist spironolactone. Large volume paracentesis or perhaps TIPPS should be considered for resistant ascites

A2

a **False**

Although a common duct stone causes jaundice it is not usually associated with confusion and disorientation. Which more strongly suggests hepatic failure

b **True**

One should not wait for toxicology levels to come back before considering this treatment. Some centres advocate the use of this agent in all causes of fulminant hepatic failure

c **False**

Hypoglycemia due to impaired glucogenesis in the liver is the usual finding.

d **True**

Breakdown of protein in the colon by bacteria to produce ammonia is one of the factors thought to contribute to encephalopathy.

e **False**

Liver transplant is a very valuable treatment with >80 per cent five-year survival

A3

a **False**

Peptic ulceration is common in patients with liver disease. Endoscopy should always be performed to confirm the bleeding is from varices and not a bleeding peptic ulcer.

b **False**

Ethanolamine, a sclerosant is used to inject varices. Adrenaline is used to induce arteriolar vasoconstriction in bleeding peptic ulcer disease.

c **True**

Endoscopic therapy of bleeding gastric varices is unsatisfactory and TIPPS should be considered early

d **False**

Propranolol reduces portal pressure, reduces rebleeding and should be considered in all patients with varices

e **True**

Although banding is probably as equally effective as sclerotherapy, it is associated with fewer complications (eg ulceration/strictures) and fewer procedures are necessary

A4

a Infective causes include hepatitis B or C (Hepatitis A does not cause chronic liver disease and thus splenomegaly is not expected). Immunological causes include autoimmune hepatitis and PBC (both commoner in females). Metabolic causes such as haemochromatosis or alpha,–AT, deficiency should be considered. She is probably too old for the first presentation of Wilson's disease

b The positive ANA would suggest autoimmune hepatitis whereas the AMA would suggest PBC. This mixed antibody profile is not uncommon. Tests to clarify the diagnosis would include immunoglobulin measurement (elevated IgG in AH, elevated IgM in PBC). Measurement of the M2 antibody (specific for PBC) and a liver biopsy would confirm PBC.

c A gastroscopy should be undertaken to look for varices. Propranolol should be given if present. Specific treatment would include Ursodeoxycholic acid (12-14 mg/kg) although recent meta-analysis data shows no evidence of therapuetic benefit

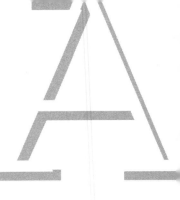

GROUP 6: Haematology and oncology

A1

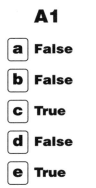

a False

b False

c True

d False

e True

Intracellular ferritin is the storage protein for iron and its synthesis parallels the amount of storage iron. A small quantity of ferritin leaves cells and circulates in the blood. In iron deficiency intracellular and serum ferritin levels are very low. Transferrin is the transport protein for iron and binds to specific receptors on erythroid precursors in the bone marrow. Receptor density is increased in iron deficiency and is reflected by an increased concentration in serum.

A fall in serum iron occurs both in iron deficiency and the anaemia of chronic disorder and cannot be used to distinguish between the two. HbA_2% is increased in beta-thalassaemia trait due to an increased synthesis of delta globin chains ($HbA_2 = (\alpha_2\delta_2)$). In iron deficiency anaemia the proportion of HbA_2 remains normal or is occasionally reduced. Serum erythropoietin is not routinely available and will be increased in most cases of anaemia from whatever cause, reflecting impaired oxygen delivery to the renal oxygen sensor.

A2

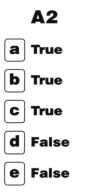

a True

b True

c True

d False

e False

Although a macrocytic anaemia is the classical presentation of pernicious anaemia, significant vitamin B_{12} deficiency can be present without anaemia and with an MCV in the normal range. Hypersegmented neutrophils will usually be present. Always check vitamin B_{12} and folate levels in patients at high risk of deficiency whether or not they have a macrocytic anaemia. Positive gastric parietal cell antibodies are a non-specific finding, and although they are usually positive in pernicious anaemia, they are also positive in large numbers of patients without pernicious anaemia. Pernicious anaemia results from gastric atrophy and failure of intrinsic factor synthesis; correction of vitamin B_{12} malabsorption by intrinsic factor in a part II Schilling test is diagnostic of pernicious anaemia, provided the patient has not had a previous partial or total gastrectomy which will produce the same result.

One injection of 1mg hydroxocobalamin IM is sufficient to produce a full haematological response. There may be an argument for repeated injections in the presence of neurological signs or symptoms. The haematological response should be monitored by following the haemoglobin concentration and reticulocyte count; failure to respond as predicted indicates additional pathology e.g. infection, iron deficiency, hypothyroidism or myelodysplasia.

A3

a She is likely to have post-transfusion purpura (PTP). This is an uncommon immunological complication of blood transfusion. Most cases are due to the presence of anti HPA-1a antibodies directed against an antigen on platelet membranes (HPA = human platelet alloantigen). It affects patients who are HPA-1a negative (approximately 1%) who as a result of previous pregnancies or blood transfusions have been immunised to the antigen. Subsequent transfusion with HPA-1a positive donor blood results in a secondary immune response, increase in the titre of anti HPA-1a and destruction of the patientís own platelets. It remains unexplained why the patientís own platelets which are HPA-1a negative are affected!

b Yes. She has headaches which might indicate intracerebral haemorrhage. Fatal intracerebral haemorrhage occurs in 10% of cases. If a platelet transfusion is given it should be from an HPA-1a negative donor; such platelets are always available at Regional Transfusion Centres.

c High dose IV immunoglobulin 0.4g/kg/24 hrs for 5 days. It is thought this works by obstruction of Fc receptors on splenic reticuloendothelial cells which are the main site of platelet destruction.

d The patient should be told she is HPA-1a negative and given a blood transfusion card stating this. Further transfusions with HPA-1a positive blood may precipitate a further episode of PTP and she should tell any future doctors looking after her that she needs HPA-1a negative blood.

A4

a Drug induced neutropenia

Normal ethnic variant

Intercurrent viral illness

Haematological malignancy

Drug toxicity should be considered in all cases of neutropenia or thrombocytopenia. Carbimazole occasionally results in agranulocytosis (<1% patients) usually early in the course of treatment. Afro-Caribbeans have a lower normal range for the neutrophil count compared with Caucasians, down to $1.0 \times 10^9/l$, but have a normal response to bacterial infection. An intercurrent viral infection may depress their neutrophil count further, down to levels normally associated with an increased risk of sepsis. The possibility of an underlying acute leukaemia or lymphoma should be borne in mind.

b Admit to hospital

Blood cultures x 2

Throat swab

MSU

CXR

Review blood film

Bone marrow aspiration

Treat with IV antibiotics

Viral serology

The patient should be admitted because she is febrile with possible drug induced neutropenia. A search for evidence of viral or bacterial infection should be undertaken. The blood film and bone marrow should be examined for the presence of blast cells or abnormal lymphoid cells. Marrow examination will exclude a haematological malignancy and, in the case of carbimazole induced neutropenia, will show reduced granulopoiesis with only occasional pro-myelocytes and little evidence of any further differentiation, so called ìmaturation arrestî.

The patient should be treated with broad spectrum IV antibiotics, modified in the light of any culture sensitivities. Consult the microbiology department for local policies on the treatment of neutropenic fever. Institute mouth care and consider prophylaxis with nystatin suspension or fluclonazole. Failure to respond or clinical deterioration should prompt the use of recombinant G-CSF which will accelerate granulopoietic recovery.

A5

a **False**

Group O Rh(D) negative blood can be provided quickly. In an emergency, before the patient's ABO and Rh(D) group is known it is the product of choice. However, supplies are very limited and ABO Rh(D) group compatible blood should be substituted as soon as the patient's ABO and Rh(D) group is known. The use of group O Rh(D) negative blood is not without risk; haemolytic transfusion reactions can still occur due to undetected antibodies against Rh antigens other than D and any other red cell antigens.

b **False**

Major transfusion reactions usually result from pre- or post analytic errors:

transposition of samples when the blood is taken

misidentification of patient when the sample is taken or the blood given

c **False**

The use of FFP should be determined by the results of repeated coagulation screens performed before and after plasma infusion

d **False**

Febrile transfusion reactions are due to antibodies to HLA or granulocyte antigens. Leucocyte depleted blood products are now available which abolish these reactions and should be used in all future transfusions

A6

a Alcohol. Either direct alcohol toxicity to megakaryocyte maturation or chronic liver disease leading to splenomegaly and hypersplenism

Intercurrent viral illness. Although the severity of the thrombocytopenia is exceptional for this mechanism

Folate deficiency. This is common in alcoholics and would account for the increased MCV

Drug toxicity. Quinine is commonly prescribed for night cramps and may result in drug dependent immune thrombocytopenia.

Haematological malignancy. Suggested by splenomegaly, macrocytosis, thrombocytopenia and leucopenia in a febrile patient

ITP. Immunological platelet destruction. Common cause of severe, acute thrombocytopenia

b Increased numbers of megakaryocytes

Normal erythroid and granulocyte maturation

ITP is due to increased peripheral consumption of platelets secondary to immunological destruction. The bone marrow responds by increasing platelet production but in all other respects is entirely normal.

c ITP. Either primary or secondary (SLE, CLL, NHL)

Drug related. Quinine, heparin induced thrombocytopenic purpura (HITT)

Infection. Viruses in general, EBV and HIV in particular. Also malaria

Post transfusion purpura (PTP)

d Lupus anti-coagulant

e Local control – nasal packing

Group and save and establish IV access

Start oral prednisolone – 60mg/day

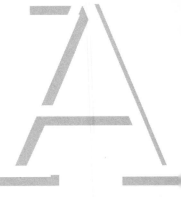

Start IV immunoglobulin ñ 0.4g/kg/24 hours

Consider blood transfusion

Consider platelet transfusion for severe, intractable haemorrhage

A7

Associated renal or liver disease

Persistent, prolonged bleeding

The presence of purpura and oozing from venepuncture sites

A8

a Isolated decrease in the fibrinogen concentration. An acquired decrease in fibrinogen due to liver disease or DIC would always be accompanied by other abnormalities. Inherited disorders usually only result in prolongation of either the PT or the APTT; abnormalities in both suggest multiple clotting factor deficiencies

b Intravascular formation of fibrin with consequent activation of the fibrinolytic system and breakdown of fibrin by plasmin

c DIC – accompanied by consumption of clotting factors and platelets with an increase in the PT and APTT, decreased fibrinogen concentration and thrombocytopenia

Extensive intravascular thrombosis with otherwise normal coagulation profile and platelet count

Liver disease – failure of hepatic clearance of fibrin D-dimers normally generated at a low rate

A9

Therapeutic heparin

Lupus anti coagulant

Acquired factor VIII inhibitor

A10

a FBC – anaemia with a reticulocytosis

Blood film – sickled red cells, polychromasia

LFT's – raised bilirubin

Sickle solubility test – positive

CAM electrophoresis – single band of Hb S

b Clinical jaundice is a feature of chronic haemolytic anaemia and although it varies in intensity, is a normal feature of HbSS. Patients with chronic anaemia have a high cardiac output and commonly have cardiomegaly with a systolic flow murmur. Splenomegaly, however, is not a feature of older children and adults with HbSS; the spleen is enlarged in infancy but atrophies due to repeated sickle cell related infarcts.

c No. This patient is unwell with a fever and splenomegaly. A patient with HbSS who is unwell but not in pain may have a serious sickle cell related complication or be unwell from any other cause.

d Splenic sequestration. Rapid pooling of blood in the spleen which often results in signs of hypovolaemia and maybe associated with pneumococcal sepsis.

Malaria. He is febrile and has recently come from a malarial region.

Persistent raised HbF. Continued gamma globin gene activity with HbF levels > 10% may ameliorate the effects of HbS, protect the spleen from infarction and result in preservation of an enlarged spleen.

e The Hb concentration is too low; most patients have a Hb of 7.0 – 9.0 g/dl in the steady state. In addition the reticulocyte count is inappropriately low suggesting an inadequate marrow response to the low haemoglobin

Thrombocytopenia is not a feature of steady state sickle cell anaemia, although it may be compatible with the patients enlarged spleen. An enlarged spleen from any cause may be associated with hypersplenism.

f Species of malaria

Parasite count

Life stage of parasite in the blood

The species is one determinant of the clinical severity of malaria; most deaths occur with Plasmodium falciparum. Speciation is based on parasite morphology or increasingly on the results of malaria antigen tests, eg Parasite F

The parasitaemia gives an indication of the parasite load and hence of clinical severity

In *Plasmodium falciparum* infection, the presence of pre-schizonts is a risk factor for cerebral malaria

g Bone marrow suppression probably mediated by increased TNF production

Hypersplenism secondary to splenomegaly

Increased haemolysis secondary to lysis of infected RBCs

Folate deficiency is common in patients from Africa with sickle cell anaemia

h Young children with sickle cell trait (HbA + HbS) with the carrier state are partially protected against dying from *Plasmodium falciparum*, but can still become infected. Patients with sickle cell anaemia (HbSS) do not have 'double protection' but can develop severe anaemia and sickle cell complications during malaria infection. Malaria is a frequent cause of death in children with sickle cell anaemia living in Africa.

A11

a Life-long

b 3.5

c International normalised ratio = PT patient's plasma/ PT control plasma[ISI]

The time for a fibrin clot to form in vitro following the addition of thromboplastin and calcium to citrate anti-coagulated plasma is recorded in seconds. This 'prothrombin time' is sensitive to the concentration of clotting factors in the extrinsic and final common pathway (II, VII, X) and is therefore used to monitor warfarin therapy, where the synthesis of factors II, VII, IX and X is impaired. The prothrombin time will also vary according to the potency of the thromboplastin used in the test; to correct for this the prothrombin time is expressed as a ratio, patient's plasma: normal control plasma, this is then adjusted by the international sensitivity index (ISI) which converts the potency of each individual thromboplastin to that of an international standard thromboplastin

d

	INR Change
Omission of doses or incorrect doses taken	↑ or ↓
Changes in diet with variation in vitamin K intake	↑ or ↓
Increase in alcohol intake	↑
Changes in concurrent drug therapy leading to changes in protein binding or liver metabolism of warfarin	↑ or ↓

e Rifampicin induces liver enzymes which increase the rate at which warfarin is metabolised and therefore reduces the anti-coagulant effect and the INR for a given dose of warfarin.

Arrange more frequent estimation of the INR and increase the dose of warfarin to maintain the INR within the therapeutic range.

f The patient had stopped anti-tuberculous chemotherapy after six months but had not attended for regular INR checks. The rate of warfarin metabolism had returned to pre-treatment levels and the degree of anti-coagulation had increased progressively.

g 5mg vitamin K IV plus prothrombin complex concentrate (50u/kg)

Vitamin K alone will have no effect on the INR for several hours and full correction may take several days. Life threatening haemorrhage requires replacement of coagulation factors. Prothrombin complex concentrate, if available, is the most effective way of achieving this but FFP, in sufficient volume (at least 1.0l) would be an alternative. The INR must be checked after infusion to confirm adequate correction, <1.8 for neurosurgery.

h Too little (<2mg) will act too slowly and produce inadequate correction, too much (> 5mg) will result in a prolonged period of warfarin resistance and a risk of valve thrombosis

A12

Marrow infiltration by abnormal plasma cells

Bleeding (eg GIT) due to thrombocytopenia from marrow infiltration or abnormal platelet function related to paraprotien

Chronic DIC - any malignancy

Anaemia of chronic disease

Diminished erythropoietin production secondary to renal failure or decreased sensitivity to erythropoietin

Poor nutrition

Chemotherapy induced myelosuppression

Microangiopathic haemolytic anaemia (any cancer)

Myeloma is a B cell neoplasm (plasma cells) that infiltrate the bone marrow, produce monoclonal immunoglobulin and free light chains (a small proportion are non-secretory). Bone destruction and renal failure are common features. DIC/microangiopathic anaemias may be seen in any malignancy (as well as in other situations eg infection). Blood loss anaemia should not be forgotten, and the anaemia of chronic disease is very common in myeloma and other malignant disorders.

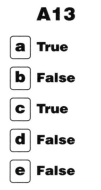

A13

a	True
b	False
c	True
d	False
e	False

Secondary polycythaemia is associated with increased Epo production and is generally seen in patients with chronic (hypoxic) lung disease, cyanotic heart disease or high altitude acclimatisation where the rise in Hb is appropriate or in patients with renal tumours where the rise in Hb serves no purpose.

Splenomegaly or an elevated platelet count are features suggestive of a primary bone marrow disorder, such as polycythaemia vera. The red cell mass is elevated in primary and secondary polycythaemia (cf spurious polycythaemia where the plasma volume is reduced). Down's syndrome has no bearing on the patient's polycythaemic state. A raised urate is more suggestive of primary polycythaemia and reflects increased DNA turnover.

A14

a	False
b	True
c	False
d	False
e	False

Characteristic implies that the features are present in most cases. Leucocytosis is sometimes found but this represents the minority of cases. Survival is long but these lymphomas are incurable, even with intensive therapies. Haemolytic anaemia may be seen but again, in the minority of cases. Chromosomal abnormalities do occur but are seldom diagnostic (most centres in the UK do not carry out chromosomal studies on marrow or blood since the translocations/deletions found are largely non-specific – unlike acute leukaemia where translocations may be diagnostic for specific subtypes of leukaemia).

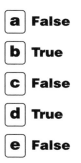

A15

a False

b True

c False

d True

e False

The majority of patients with acute leukaemia have chromosomal abnormalities (not all are detected using standard cytogenetic analysis). Some abnormalities are characteristic of specific leukaemic subtypes eg t(15;17) in AML M3, (acute promyelocytic leukaemia), inv (16) in AML M4, t(8;21) in AML M2. Other abnormalities such as the Philadelphia chromosome t(9;22) while common in CML may also be found in ALL and so are not entirely specific. Some karyotypic abnormalities are associated with good prognosis eg t(8;21), t(15;17) but complex or evolving chromosomal abnormalities typically characterise poor prognostic groups.

CML and other myeloproliferations may be associated with hyperuricaemia and gout due to high cell turnover. Myelodysplastic syndromes are primary marrow disorders characterised by ineffective haemopoiesis, hypercellular bone marrow and blood cytopenias. Paraprotein production is seldom found. Alkylating agents such as chlorambucil or cyclophosphamide are associated with development of secondary malignancies five-to-ten years later including acute leukaemia.

A16

Take a full history and examine patient. Check for bruising, lymphadenopathy, hepatosplenomegaly, gum hypertrophy, fever, pallor. Ask about blood loss (especially menstrual), previous anaemia, drug ingestion, sweats, anorexia, weight loss, recent infection (and foreign travel).

Arrange FBC and blood film examination. Check haematinics (B12, folate, ferritin). Biochemistry screen - generally checked but probably won't add much. Monospot/Paul Bunnell for infective mononucleosis. If generalised lymphodenopathy consider biopsy and bone marrow aspirate/trephine biopsy.

In general, after taking the history, examining the patient and performing the FBC, the cause for the patient's anaemia should be fairly obvious. This patient had been well but latterly felt tired. She had no history of infection, her appetite was good and her weight steady. FBC confirmed the WCC and platelets were normal. The MCV was reduced (70fl) and blood film was normal apart from RBC microcytosis.

Serum ferritin was reduced confirming iron deficiency anaemia. Her lymphadenopathy was confined to the inguinal regions (<1cm diameter) and was felt to be benign.

If node biopsy is needed, avoid biopsying inguinal glands since they often show reactive changes; cervical/axillary nodes are more useful for diagnosis of lymphoma.

A17

a False

b False

c False

d False

e False

Differentiating between reactive thrombocytosis and primary (essential) thrombocythaemia is often very difficult since no single test exists that is diagnostic of ET. This man's elevated WCC may reflect an underlying disease/infection or be part of his myeloproliferative state, and does not help us to define the cause. The spleen is more likely to be enlarged in ET than reactive causes. Karyotypic analysis in reactive thrombocytosis will be normal, but is also likely to be normal in ET. Burning discomfort such as this is termed erythromelalgia and is a feature of ET. Iron deficiency may be due to underlying colonic carcinoma (reactive thrombocytosis), upper GIT bleeding (inducing reactive thrombocytosis) and caused by ET, so does not help us make the diagnosis.

A18

a False

b True

c False

d False

e True

Patients who are taking corticosteroids often have an elevated WCC, but these are neutrophils; eosinophils numbers are reduced. Lymphocytosis is a feature of leukaemia (lymphoid), lymphoma, viral infection and some bacterial infections (pertussis, brucellosis) and TB. Toxic granulation of neutrophils occurs in a variety of disorders - infective, inflammatory, trauma etc. and does not aid the diagnosis of underlying infection. If there is vascular stasis due to a high WCC the best immediate treatment is cytoreduction using a cell separator - effect is much faster than chemotherapy (hours rather than days). Following splenectomy the WCC is often elevated and may return to normal after weeks/months or may remain high. Platelets also rise post-splenectomy.

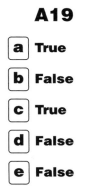

A19

a True

b False

c True

d False

e False

In chronic blood loss the MCV falls when the patient develops iron deficiency, but following a brisk bleed the MCV (and Hb initially) will remain normal. Thalassaemias are characterised by reduced MCV and thalassaemia trait is no exception. In sickle cell disease there are marked RBC morphological abnormalities but the MCV is normal. Severe, acute haemolysis may be associated with an increased MCV; reticulocytes are slightly larger than mature red blood cells. Folate deficiency and alcoholism result in a macrocytic anaemia. Alcohol excess is the commonest cause for a macrocytosis, thought to be related to alterations in red cell membrane lipids. Alcoholism may be complicated by folate deficiency; the MCV may increase further and erythropoiesis in the bone marrow will be megaloblastic.

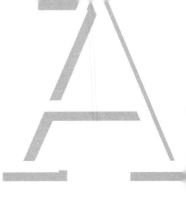

GROUP 7: Geriatrics

A1

All elderly patients should have multidisciplinary assessment. The supervising PHYSICIAN would assess and treat the underlying medical and mental problems as appropriate. He or she should comment on the prognosis.

The PHYSIOTHERAPIST would assess the patient's functional abilities and the potential for further improvement. He or she should also comment on the patient's progress.

The OCCUPATIONAL THERAPIST would look at the patient's abilities to care for him or herself, arrange a home visit if necessary, and also arrange the necessary alterations and amendments.

The SOCIAL WORKER would arrange the necessary help needed at home, and ensure the carer visits the patient regularly and reports back should any problems arise.

The DISTRICT NURSE's role is to deliver the medical treatment as needed eg dressing of ulcers, insulin injections etc.

The above team, which may include the speech therapist and dietician, should meet and discuss the case at least once a week while the patient remains in hospital.

A2

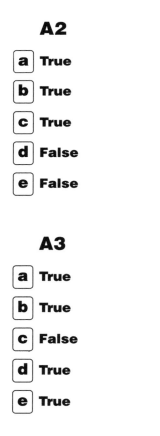

a True

b True

c True

d False

e False

A3

a True

b True

c False

d True

e True

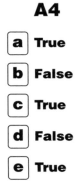

A4

a True

b False

c True

d False

e True

A5

a Whether his wife witnessed the fall and if so, the circumstances of the fall and whether he lost consciousness. Memory of loss of consciousness is not a reliable guide to the actual events. If laceration has been present it is important not to miss 'dirty' wounds, eg falls in the garden, which might need tetanus prophylaxis.

b FBC for anaemia/sepsis - underlying causes of falls

U&E, creatinine, glucose for dehydration - cause of fall or consequence

Consider CPK if extensive bruising, or long period of time on the floor after falling

CXR and ECG for causes of falls

Pelvic X-rays and hip X-ray for fractures

c He should be assessed for MI by serial cardiac enzymes (including CK MB fraction as CK alone is likely to be raised due to fall). His fall is possibly related to bradycardia, and as long as he is on no drugs likely to slow his rate, (eg Digoxin), he should be considered for cardiac pacing.

A6

a True

These are a common cause of OH, and even in the presence of hypertension, a drop of BP on standing can be significant and symptomatic

b False

Although drugs are a common cause, some patients develop OH with no other disease process or medication. These patients can benefit from advice and occasionally therapy with fludrocortisone

c False

Caffeine containing drinks should be encouraged as they increase BP, but not more that five cups of coffee or strong tea a day

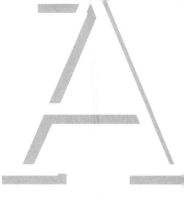

d **False**

Pacing does not help OH unless underlying bradyarrhythmias

e **True**

Co-existent sepsis is an important cause of OH, dehydration and vasodilatation

A7

a **True**

Temporary focal neurological signs are common after fits in the elderly

b **True**

c **False**

This is more suggestive of cardiac cause, although not a 'hard' sign

d **False**

A normal EEG does not rule out epilepsy, and if clinical suspicion is high, treatment should still be instituted

e **True**

Most new onset epilepsy in the elderly is caused by vascular disease, either multi-infarct or strokes

A8

a Previous ischaemic heart disease, drug history, contraindications to thrombolysis, in particular whether he has proliferative diabetic retinopathy

b In the absence of contraindications, treatment with thrombolysis and aspirin should be instituted. If he was not breathless by his mild LVF diuretics may be withheld initially to reduce the risk of underfilling in acute MI

c Secondary prevention should be started with an ACE inhibitor. In most elderly patients, ACE inhibitors are more suitable than ß blockers post MI. All should receive aspirin unless contraindicated

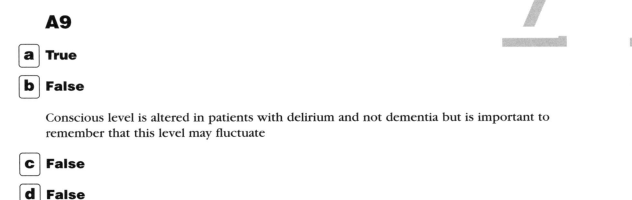

A9

a True

b False

Conscious level is altered in patients with delirium and not dementia but is important to remember that this level may fluctuate

c False

d False

e True

Short-term memory impairment is an early and salient feature of dementia

A10

Drugs

Electrolytes/Endocrine disturbance

Drug withdrawal

Infections

Reduced sensory input

Intracranial problems

Urinary retention/faecal impaction

Myocardial ischaemia, arrhythmias, CHF

A11

a True

b False

Geriatric Depression Scale is a screening test, not a diagnostic test

c True

d True

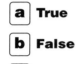

A12

a True

b False

c False

Only some patients with mild to moderate dementia of Alzheimer's type respond to donepezil, an acetyl choline transferase inhibitor

d True

e True

A13

Hypothyroidism

B_{12} deficiency

Folate deficiency

Hypoglycaemia

Alcohol

Depression

Sub-dural haematoma

Normal pressure hydrocephalus

A14

a True

History from GP would be helpful particularly in relation to the patient's previous mental state as dementia is a risk factor for delirium

b True

c True

d False

e False

f True

History and examination support the diagnosis of delirium caused by chest infection.
Therefore chest X-Ray would be helpful in confirming the diagnosis

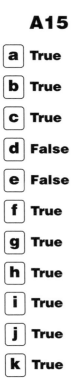

g False

A15

a True

b True

c True

d False

e False

f True

g True

h True

i True

j True

k True

A16

a True

b True

c True

d False

e True

Neck stiffness and rigidity of limbs can be noted in patients with hypothermia of 29-30°C.
This may be associated with flapping tremor

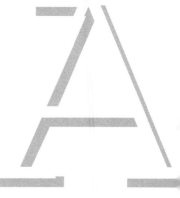

A17

a True

b True

c True

d True

Vascular thromboses and ventricular fibrillation are likely to arise in patients with severe hypothermia

Cardiac arrhythmias may also be produced by rapid rewarming

A18

a True

b True

c True

d True

e True

f False

g False

h False

Although blood should be taken for thyroid function tests at time of admission, the measurement can be carried out at a later stage, unless hypothyroidism is considered in the initial diagnosis

A19

a FBC

U&E

LFT

TFT

Chest X-ray

ECG

MSU – culture and dipstick

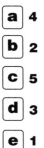

b Urinary tract infection

c Silent myocardial ischaemia/infarction (subendocardial)

A20

a 4

b 2

c 5

d 3

e 1

A21

Hypertension

Smoking

AF

Diabetes

A22

a Left Atrium in AF

b Heart valves in infective endocarditis

c Atheromatous neck vessels

A23

False

A24

Cerebral abscess

Subdural haematoma

Sub arachnoid haemorrhage

Epileptic fit

Hypoglycaemia

A25

Aspiration pneumonia

PE

Pressure sores

Depression

A26

False

A27

False

A28

Futility/ineffectiveness

Patient's wishes

Justice

Quality of life

A29

[a] **False**

Tremor occurs in 70 per cent of patients at presentation

b **True**

Arteriosclerotic Parkinsonism occurs more commonly in patients with hypertension and cerebrovascular disease

c **False**

Major tranquillisers, particularly depot preparations, are the commonest cause

d **False**

Parkinson's disease is a clinical diagnosis

A30

Gout

Pseudogout

Septic arthritis

Haemarthrosis

Acute flare up of chronic arthritis

A31

True

A32

Joint aspiration – fluid for culture/fluid for crystals

Blood cultures

Serum uric acid

X-ray of joint

ESR, WCC

A33

a Colchicine or prednisolone; non-steroidal anti-inflammatory drugs would worsen heart failure and should be avoided

b Diclofenac and misoprostol; indomethacin; methyl prednisolone injection; lignocaine injection

c Benzyl penicillin; flucloxacillin; gentamicin; plus diclofenac and misoprostol or indomethacin

A34

True

Urate crystals are negatively birefringent.

A35

False

25-32mmHg

A36

Ill elderly people

Patients undergoing surgery

Patients with neurological disease including spinal cord injury

Patients having palliative care

A37

To monitor severity and progress of the wound

Medicolegal requirements as litigation may arise

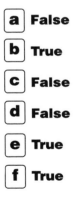

A38

a True

b True

c False

d False

e True

A39

Poor nutritional state

Low body weight

Motor deficiency

Sensory deficit

Intercurrent illness

Incontinence

A40

a False

b True

c False

d False

e True

f True

A41

To look for osteomyelitis

A42

a | **True**

The risks of anticoagulation due to poor compliance, falls, etc, make this inappropriate

b | **False**

Patients up to 85 can benefit from anticoagulation with reduced risk of stroke, but they should be carefully selected

c | **True**

d | **False**

ACE inhibition may be useful in patients to control heart failure, but renal function and BP should be monitored closely

e | **True**

A43

a | **False**

Antibiotics should be started after stix testing, but results of culture not awaited

b | **False**

Resistance is very rare (look up figures)

c | **False**

Although UTI can cause incontinence through bladder instability, most patients with incontinence do not have UTI, and in the absence of stix positivity to leucocytes or nitrites, antibiotics are not indicated

d | **False**

Catheterisation should be avoided as it carries higher risks of infection and septicaemia

e | **False**

Residual volume of up to 100ml can be considered normal

A44

a | To examine and investigate for acute or remediable medical precipitants to the admission

b | Phone duty social worker The duty social worker could organise appropriate emergency accommodation in a residential home while the reasons for discharge failure are investigated and appropriate long term plans made

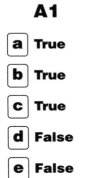

GROUP 8: Rheumatology

A1

a True

b True

c True

d False

e False

The main diseases in seronegative spondyloarthropathies include ankylosing spondylitis, arthritis associated with inflammatory bowel disease, psoriatic arthritis, reactive arthritis and Reiter's disease (reactive arthritis: reactive to infective diarrhoea and genitourinary infection such as gonorrhoea/chlamydia)

A2

a False

The classical deformities, ie ulnar deviation, Boutonnière's and swan neck are late manifestations

b True

Vertical subluxation is less common than atlantoaxial subluxation but has a higher mortality rate due to movement of the odontoid peg up into the foramen magnum

c False

Disease modifying agents are used early to prevent erosions

d False

Seronegative RA is well described

e True

Any synovitis of the wrist may lead to carpal tunnel syndrome

A3

a **True**

Ankylosing spondylitis is associated with HLA B27 and may be a feature of psoriatic arthritis

b **False**

The common patterns include asymmetrical DIP joint disease and a lower limb oligoarthritis

c **True**

d **False**

There is no correlation between the two

e **True**

So does methotrexate and to a lesser extent azathioprine

A4

a **True**

But true inflammatory arthritis/synovitis is rare

b **False**

cANCA with specificity proteins for proteinase 3 is a very sensitive marker for Wegener's granulomatosis (WG)

c **True**

Also includes facial pain, nose bleeds and deafness

d **True**

Mononeuritis multiplex usually has a vasculitic basis

e **False**

Cyclophosphamide together with steroids has improved the five year survival from 20 per cent to 90 per cent

A5

a **True**

The treatment of Hepatitis B positive PAN includes plasma exchange and antiviral agents

b **False**

Pulmonary involvement is rare in PAN. Microscopic polyangiitis as Wegener's granulomatosis may be complicated by pulmonary haemorrhage

c **True**

Visceral infarction (liver, spleen, bowel and kidney) is characteristic

d **True**

Often a mononeuritis multiplex

e **False**

Usually renal infarction, not glomerulonephritis

A6

a **False**

Lupus profundus is rare. It is a form of panniculitis that leads to subcutaneous fat atrophy

b **True**

Especially in the presence of antiphospholipid antibodies

c **False**

There is no diagnostic test for lupus cerebritis. MRI and CSF examination should be performed to exclude other pathology

d **True**

Sm antibodies are rare (5 – 10% of SLE) but when present are the most specific autoantibody

e **True**

Neonatal lupus syndrome occurs in 1-5% of Ro positive mothers. It may consist of cholestatic jaundice and a widespread discoid rash in the new-born infant. These are self limiting. Complete congenital heart block is irreversible and may develop at around 20 weeks gestation

A7

a **False**

RA virtually never initially presents with knee synovitis

b **True**

Gout and pseudogout are the likeliest

c **True**

Gout and pseudogout are the likeliest

d **False**

This is not known to cause knee swelling

e **False**

This is not known to cause knee swelling

A8

a **False**

The full histological picture is acinar destruction, duct dilation and florid lymphocytic infiltration with plasma cells

b **True**

Less than 5mm of wetness of the paper after 5 minutes is indicative of reduced tear production

c **True**

Usually vasculitic in origin; vasculitis of the vasa nervosum

d **True**

Cryoglobulins are usually composed of IgM rheumatoid factors. These behave like large immune complexes and result in vasculitis

e **False**

Ro and La antibodies are common but not universal

A9

a **False**

Involvement of the first carpometacarpal joint at the thumb base is characteristic and leads to the 'square hand' appearance of OA

b **True**

Twin studies have identified a strong genetic component to nodal OA

c **False**

Heberden's/Bouchard's nodes not Oslers

d **False**

Patients with OA are usually obese and at low risk for osteoporosis. In contrast, thin women are at risk for osteoporosis but not OA. The reasons for this dichotomy are unclear

e **False**

If the metacarpophalangeal joints are involved, inflammatory arthritis, e.g. RA or psoriatic arthritis is more likely

A10

a **False**

Early mobilisation/physiotherapy leads to quicker resolution of symptoms

b **False**

Lasègue's (sciatic stretch test) is useful when positive, but is not always positive

c **True**

Schmorl's node is usually asymptomatic

d **False**

L5/S1 is the commonest, followed by L4/5 level

e **False**

MRI scanning is usually only considered if surgery is being contemplated. The vast majority of simple mechanical disc lesions are self limiting and do not need imaging at all

A11

a **False**

PMR is the classically insidious presentation of a rheumatic disease

b **True**

Known as polymyalgic onset of RA. Both PMR and RA are commonly associated with HLA DR4

c **True**

Monthly im methylprednisone injections have been shown in a randomised study to be an effective treatment for PMR that is equal to low dose prednisone 7.5mg daily but with fewer corticosteroid adverse effects

d **True**

Ultrasound studies show a high prevalence of shoulder effusions in PMR

e **True**

Bence Jones protein analysis and a protein strip should be considered in all patients presenting with PMR-like symptoms

A12

a **True**

A recent study in the BMJ suggests this

b **False**

Alcohol intake, moderate or excessive increases the risk of osteoporosis, as does smoking

c **True**

Self explanatory

d **True**

The T score rather than the Z score is a good predictor of fracture risk

e **True**

Also vertebral and hip fractures

A13

a | True

May rapidly lead to renal failure

b | True

Pulmonary renal vasculitic syndromes include : Wegener's granulomatosis, Churg Strauss syndrome, microscopic polyangiitis and Goodpasture's (anti GBM) disease

c | True

pANCA recognises myeloperoxidase and a few other neutrophil enzymes

d | True

Pulmonary haemorrhage is characteristic of microscopic polyangiitis and Wegener's granulomatosis

e | True

Corneal melts, scleritis, episcleritis and retinal vasculitis are all features of Wegener's granulomatosis

A14

Subcutaneous calcinosis, Raynaud's, oesophagitis, sclerodactyly and telangiectasiae may be features of the CREST syndrome; a variant of systematic sclerosis

Other features:

Cardiac: Pericarditis, myocarditis, hypertension

Pulmonary: Interstitial lung disease/pulmonary fibrosis, pulmonary hypertension, pleural effusion, pleuritic chest pain

GI: dysphagia, small bowel and large bowel disease, malabsorption, diverticulae, perforation. reflux oesophagitis

Renal: Hypertensive renal crisis, leading to renal failure

Joint: Polyarthralgia, occasionally synovitis

Autoantibodies: Anti centromere, a good prognostic marker associated with 'CREST' variant

Anti Scl70 (DNA topoisomerase I)

Anti RNA polymerase I & III (Both these are poor prognostic indicators associated with more diffuse disease)

GROUP 9: Renal

A1

a Volume depletion/Hypotension/Haemorrhage

LVF/sympathetic overdrive

(Vasospasm/Raynaud's/Cold)

b Increased JVP

Increased BP

Fourth heart sound/gallop rhythm

No postural drop

c Total body salt & water overload

d Peripheral pulses palpable

Vascular bruits (femoral, carotid)

Abdominal bruits

Decreased postural BP

All to try and clinically exclude renal artery stenosis

e Ultrasound or isotope renogram (NOT angiography)

f Ultrasound

 - Unequal renal size

 - Aortic aneurysm

Renogram

 - Unequal divided function

 - Unequal perfusion phase

 - Bilateral poor perfusion

 - Unequal size

 - Delayed transit time

A2

a Fluid depletion/pre-renal uraemia/volume depletion (Diagnosis 1)

Multi-system vasculitis/rapidly progressive GN (uncontrolled sepsis) (Diagnosis 2)

b Urine dipstick (for protein and blood); urine microscopy (for red cell casts)

c **Diagnosis 1**

– Falling weight

– decreased JVP/tachycardia

Diagnosis 2

– Splinter haemorrhages/nail fold infarcts/mononeuritis multiplex/vasculitic rash

d Worsening pulmonary haemorrhage precipitated by pulmonary oedema

(worsening sepsis)

e ABG

CVP line

ITU/Nephrology referral

Blood cultures

A3

a Insert a urine catheter. Urine retention must not be missed as its immediate management is so straight forward

b If a patient is anuric you still must consider obstruction, and in this case it could be above the level of the bladder. Arrange for an ultrasound

A4

a You can't! The surgery planned is routine and the patient is asymptomatic. If the patient had neurological features of severe cerebral oedema then closely supervised use of 2N saline plus diuretics is indicated

b An assessment of fluid status is essential. In this case the examination is normal. The most likely diagnosis is SIADH where you will find a low serum osmolarity associated with an inappropriately low urine osmolarity

c Restrict fluid intake and assess fluid status regularly. Daily weight is an essential tool

A5

a Assess fluid status and don't be afraid to replace fluid losses. In CRF the renal response to Na^+ and water loss is blunted and the patient can become severely dehydrated

Giving IV fluids will create a potentially vicious circle.

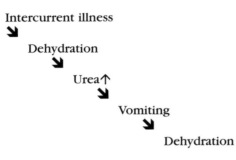

Intercurrent illness
↘
    Dehydration
    ↘
        Urea↑
        ↘
           Vomiting
           ↘
              Dehydration

b Central line (but avoid subclavian) to optimise fluid management

Renal tract imaging – remember you cannot afford to miss an obstruction

GROUP 10: Cardiology

A1

a | Supine valsalva manoeuvre

Intravenous adenosine

Intravenous digoxin may be dangerous as the conduction though the AV node may be slowed whilst the conduction through the extra pathway would be increased. Intravenous amiodarone would only be appropriate after failure of adenosine, vagal manoeuvres and recurrence after DC shock. DC cardioversion would be appropriate after failure of supine valsalva manoeuvre and intravenous adenosine

b | Referred for electrophysiological study

The patient has WPW Syndrome; an EP study is definitive and assesses risk of rapid conduction in AF which is potentially fatal. Referral for 24 hour tape would not be of much value unless symptoms are very frequent. Digoxin may aggravate WPW symptoms and although amiodarone is effective it is now outdated in era of R/F ablation. Referral for an echocardiogram is not indicated as WPW not usually associated with structural heart disease.

A2

a | Urea & electrolytes

Urinary cortisol

Likely to be related to oral contraceptive pill. Minimal investigation needed

b | Urea & electrolytes (to exclude renal disease/Conn's)

ECG (to stratify risk)

FBC (macrocytosis is evidence of alcohol excess)

LFT (evidence of alcohol excess)

Likely to be essential HT possibly aggravated by alcohol intake

c | Renal ultrasound

Isotope renogram

Need to exclude significant renovascular disease

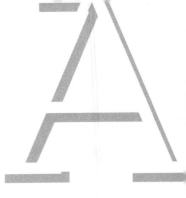

|d| Urinary/plasma catecholamines

Urinary cortisol

Plasma renin/aldosterone levels

CT abdomen

Strong possibility of secondary cause, especially Conn's syndrome

A3

|a| IV diamorphine for rapid symptom relief and pulmonary vasodilation

IV/buccal nitrate for rapid reduction in venous return plus arteriolar dilation. (Buccal route is cheaper and as quick)

IV frusemide as IV diuretics have some haemodynamic as well as diuretic effect. Oral diuretics may not be well absorbed initially

Oral digoxin. This is absorbed rapidly (IV may be used if patient vomiting)

Oral diuretic. Initial doses of diuretics tend to be high to clear oedema and can often be adjusted downwards when patient is stable

Oral ACEI. Start after acute situation is over and titrate to a high dose assuming no contraindication

A4

|a| Acute myocardial infarction

Aortic dissection

Pericarditis

Oesophageal pain

|b| Was the pain sudden (instantaneous)? If yes – increases the likelihood of aortic dissection, as does back pain

Is the pain worse on movement/respiration? If yes – increases the likelihood of pericarditis, musculoskeletal pain or pleurisy

Is the pain related to posture? If yes – increases the possibility of oesophageal pain

Is the pain associated with sweating or nausea? If yes – makes pericarditis and oesophageal pain less likely

c ECG – remember it may also be normal in early stages of a myocardial infarction and at all stages of a dissection

Chest X-ray – look for mediastinal widening to suggest a dissection

CT/MRI – if available locally. If not arrange an echo or if dissection strongly suspected refer to cardiac centre.

A5

a Give IV lignocaine. SVT with aberration very unlikely in known CHD

Arrange cardioversion – the sooner, the better!

Blood for U & E – hypokalaemia may be important

b Continue IV lignocaine

Assess cardiac status – is there evidence of heart failure as a precipitant

CXR – evidence of pulmonary congestion

Blood for cardiac enzymes – if VT is due to a 'silent' MI the prognosis is much better than for a primary arrhythmia

c Beta blockers: particularly suitable in CHD. Sotalol may have advantages over other beta blockers

Amiodarone: very effective but has long term side effects

Other anti-arrhythmics: relatively contra-indicated in CHD due to risk of pro-arrhythmia

Further investigation:

Electrophysiological studies may indicate need for implantable defibrillator

Angiography in case of critical ischaemia as a contributory cause

A6

a Aspirin, statin, beta blockers. Generally falls in good prognosis group; benefit of beta blockers marginal

b Aspirin, ACEI, beta blockers. Beta blockers of particular benefit in this group (in addition to ACEI) if they can be tolerated. Start fibrate or statin as necessary once lipid profile established

c Aspirin, beta blockers, ACEI. At this age anterior MI likely to be associated with significant LV dysfunction despite absence of heart failure and ACEI is indicated. A statin would be indicated if high cholesterol is found

d ACEI, statin. No evidence exists for antiplatelet agents other than aspirin, but could consider dipyridamole, or clopidogrel; warfarin is an alternative. Verapamil and diltiazem contraindicated if there has been any evidence of heart failure

e Aspirin, nitrate/hydralazine, warfarin indicated for secondary prevention of thrombo embolism with AF in the presence of heart failure and prior HT, but may have value for CHD too. Can be co-prescribed fairly safely with low dose aspirin. As intolerant of ACEI, nitrate/hydralazine combination should be considered though no direct evidence of benefit in the context of acute MI as opposed to chronic heart failure.

A7

a **No**

Low BP (<100 mmHg on admission) carries a bad prognosis

b **Yes**

Raised urea carries a bad prognosis even when creatinine normal

c **Yes**

Association of acute pulmonary oedema and acute myocardial infarction can result in a hospital mortality of 50%

d **No**

Not an independent factor in prognosis

e **No**

Not an independent factor in prognosis

f **Yes**

Prior hypertension, diabetes carry worse prognosis

g **Yes**

Hyponatraemia on presentation carries a worse prognosis

h **No**

Hyperkalaemia associated with poor prognosis in heart failure

A8

a **False**

No direct correlation, in severe AS the murmur becomes softer as LV function declines

b **True**

Because the Doppler beam may not be aligned exactly with the aortic jet, significant underestimates of stenosis can occur. Always be suspicious if patient with aortic systolic murmur is symptomatic. Further investigations eg catheterisation, may be necessary.

c **False**

With the demise of rheumatic heart disease as a cause, aortic stenosis is now a disease of the elderly with a rising incidence from 60-80. Up to 5% of patients over 80 have some degree of degenerative aortic valve disease

d **False**

Aortic stenosis results in concentric LV hypertrophy, not dilation

e **True**

In the elderly a rigid arterial tree may maintain high pulse pressure despite significant aortic stenosis

A9

a **True**

In current practice valvoplasty is as effective as closed mitral valvotomy and has a lower morbidity

b **True**

Length not loudness of the diastolic murmur reflects severity

c **False**

Doppler ultrasound is reliably accurate in mitral stenosis, because it is much easier to align the beam to the flow of blood through the mitral valve than is the case for the aortic valve

d **False**

A loud first heart sound and opening snap reflect a pliant valve suitable for valvoplasty. These findings are now much less important in the era of echocadiography

e **False**

Anticoagulants are indicated in all patients with mitral valve disease and AF

A10

a Diuretics – intravenous/oral

Digoxin – especially useful in presence of gallop rhythm

Insulin – metformin relatively contra indicated in heart failure because of lactic acidosis

b Alcoholic cardiomyopathy

Ischaemic cardiomyopathy

Viral myocarditis

Severe mitral regurgitation

c Ischaemic cardiomyopathy: dilated cardiomyopathy (viral or alcoholic) usually leads to global LV dysfunction; the focal akinesia seen suggests silent ischaemic heart disease. Mitral regurgitation is clearly functional rather than the primary cause.

d Coronary angiography – to define the anatomy

Isotope perfusion scan – to identify whether there is 'hibernating' myocardium

Cardiac catheterisation confirms severe three vessel coronary disease with poor LV function. Isotope perfusion scan suggested significant 'hibernation'. Three months later on outpatient review, he is well and symptom free on digoxin diuretics, ACEI and warfarin. Elective CABG is recommended but the patient declines

Note: CABG has been shown to markedly improve survival in this high risk group with three vessel disease and impaired LV function. There is, however, a substantially increased perioperative mortality. A grey decision!

A11

a Thiazide diuretic or beta blockers: only drugs currently shown to improve long term cardiovascular risk in this age group.

b Beta blockers (atenolol or labetalol) and methyldopa. Very limited experience with any of the newer classes of drugs in pregnancy

c ACEI. Particularly valuable in preventing the progression of nephropathy in diabetics

d Dihydropyridines, ACEI, thiazide diuretic. Shown to reduce cardiovascular mortality in this group

e Verapamil/Diltiazem: useful anti-hypertensive and allow rate control during episodes of AF (though probably do not prevent occurrence of AF)

A12

a Vaso-vagal attack: common but unusual at this age without precipitating cause

b Cardiac arrhythmia: hypertension likely to be associated with heart disease.Bradycardia more likely than tachycardia

c Cough syncope: possible if significant airways obstruction

d Iatrogenic: postural hypotension from antihypertensive medication, check lying and standing blood pressure

A13

a **No**

Digoxin has no useful effect in restoring SR

b **Yes**

DC cardioversion should be undertaken if failure to respond to drug treatment

c **Yes**

Flecainide can restore SR in 50-60% of patients in this category (no underlying cardiac disease)

d **No**

Although effective, IV amiodarone is not appropriate in the short term management of AF

e **No**

Anticoagulation unnecessary where AF has been present less than 24 hours

A14

a **False**

A history of HT is a risk factor for future thrombo-embolism

b **True**

Cardiomegaly usually reflects impaired LV function, an important risk factor for thrombo-embolism

c **False**

The major risk factors for thrombo-embolism are HT, cardiac failure, and previous embolic event (especially neurological)

d **False**

Providing there are no contraindications, anti-coagulation is equally effective in the elderly

e **False**

Current recommendations are to continue anti-coagulants for at least four weeks because of the risk of relapse

A15

Analgesia – IV diamorphine

ECG – establish diagnosis and criteria for thrombolysis

Aspirin 300mg orally

Establish history and exclude contra-indications to thrombolysis

Give thrombolysis

A16

a **False**

Sudden (instantaneous) onset of pain is classical of aortic dissection and rarely occurs with MI

b **False**

Pericardial rubs can be very transient; the diagnosis depends on the history and characteristic ECG changes

c **True**

The thrombolytic trials shows an excess of cardiac rupture in the first 24 hours following thrombolysis, but this is more than offset by improved mortality over next 30 days

d **True**

Aortic dissection characteristically tears inferiorly to involve the ostium of the right coronary artery and cause a true inferior infarct. Beware: Thrombolysis contra-indicated!

e **False**

Transthoracic echo can provide suggestive evidence of aortic dissection but is often negative. Investigations of choice are trans-oesophageal echo, CT or MRI scan of the aorta

A17

a **True**

Detection of RV infarction by ST elevation in V3R-V4R in the early stages is a good way to risk stratify patients with an inferior MI

b **False**

Ventricular septal rupture causes RV overload and pulmonary oedema only presents if extensive LV damage as well

c **False**

Heart Failure at any stage is the most important determinant of long term survival. Early VF has no real long term consequences as it simply reflects acute myocardial damage

d **False**

Cardiogenic shock in acute MI is the result of myocardial stunning. Hibernation is a phenomenon seen in chronic heart failure

e **False**

Volume expansion in RV infarction is best given using IV dextrose because of the risk of pulmonary oedema if there is pre existing LV disease

f **True**

Hospital mortality in ST depression infarct, not eligible for thrombolysis is 20%, twice the average for ST elevation infarcts, which receive thrombolysis. ST depression infarcts show no benefit from thrombolysis either, and should be considered for early angiography

A18

Analgesia – IV diamorphine if oral (buccal) GTN ineffective

IV nitrates

Measure urgent fibrinogen: good measure of effectiveness of streptokinase – should be less than 1mg/dl up to 24 hours after administration

Rethrombolyse. Choice is between further streptokinase or tPa. If in doubt about streptokinase resistence (ie fibrinogen unavailable) consider tPa, but discuss with CONSULTANT in view of risk of haemorrhage

A19

a **False**

Thrombo-embolism is a feature of pacemaker patients with sick sinus syndrome and slow AF; it is not increased in complete heart block per se

b **True**

Dual chamber pacing is only needed if there is evidence of AV nodal disease as well (usually identified by pacing the atrium at 140/min during the implantation to see if heart block develops)

c **False**

Retrograde conduction is (with asynchronous atrio-ventricular contraction) a cause of the pacemaker syndrome but is seen only in single chamber ventricular pacing (eg VVI)

d **False**

No indication for pacing in the absence of symptoms, but regular follow-up required

e **False**

GROUP 11: Respiratory

A1

a False

The elevated HCO_3 indicates a degree of compensation. By correcting the pH back to normal using 1kPa CO_2 = 0.1 pH approximately, the pCO_2 is 11.6, chronic respiratory failure

b False

c False

Intubation is determined by clinical picture not ABG result. This patient may be alert and co-operative although distressed and improve rapidly with treatment

d True

Uncontrolled O_2 ie high FiO_2 in the ambulance commonly results in patients arriving semi-comatose after climbing into the ambulance 15 minutes previously. In this situation NIV is very effective and the exception to the normal rule that coma is a contraindication to NIV

A2

a False

There is no danger of CO_2 narcosis and high FiO_2 should be employed

b True

Beta-agonists may result in further hypoxaemia by increasing ventilation to poorly perfused lung ie worsening VQ

c False

Aminophylline may not even be second line treatment due to significant morbidity and relative lack of effect. There is no evidence of synergism with other bronchodilators despite the theoretical expectation that beneficial interactions would occur

d False

Sedatives should not be used in asthma

A3

a True

This may arise because of the slow rate producing alveolar hypoventilation plus impaired function of the ventilatory pump because of the flail chest

b **False**

A cause for the respiratory depression must be established first. As a head injury is possible - any epileptogenic drug is contra-indicated

c **True**

All unconscious patients should have ABG performed at triage at A&E

d **True**

If given – if not a primary cerebral injury must be assumed. The patient should be intubated and CT scanning performed (after thorough external examination of skull and external auditory meatuses).

e **False**

With O_2 therapy the oximeter might be falsely reassuring as the O_2 saturation will be normal despite potentially severe CO_2 narcosis

A4

a **False**

Large series report that the majority of causes of major haemoptysis are benign

b **True**

Assessing the lung from which bleeding is coming is important but may still be difficult at bronchoscopy as haemorrhage and clot may be widespread throughout bronchial tree

c **False**

d **True**

Although technically difficult, and with the risk of spinal cord injury as aberrant spinal vessels may arise from intercostal arteries, bronchial artery occlusion with gel foam or metalic particles is usually effective. Lung infarction rarely occurs as the lung continues to gain oxygenation from the pulmonary arteries

A5

a **True**

The demonstration of an acute respiratory alkalosis with normal A-a gradient is suggestive of hyperventilation syndrome

b **True**

Although an unusual history

c **False**

Although a V/Q scan may be appropriate to exclude recurrent thrombo-embolism it can be done when convenient not urgently

d **True**

Associated features of carpopedal spasm, generalised muscle weakness and perioral tingling would be typical of the hyperventilation syndrome and arise because of impaired myoneuronal function due to alkalosis

A6

a **True**

Bronchoconstriction induced by topical beta-blocker therapy for glaucoma is well recognised

b **False**

This is unlikely on the given history

c **True**

If the cause is asthma. Asthma may develop at any age although the peak age is in youth or early adulthood. As a minimum a CXR should be performed and serial peak flows assessed before prescribing inhaled or oral steroids

d **True**

The expiratory envelope may demonstrate a scalloped mid expiratory portion indicating pressure dependant airway collapse typical of emphysema. A truncated expiratory peak flow in combination with limited inspiratory flow rates would suggest fixed upper airway obstruction eg thyroid enlargement compressing trachea

e **False**

It may be indicated but CXR should be performed first

A7

a **False**

More likely to be polycythaemic!

b **True**

Not only would this indicate severity of COPD but also response to bronchodilator treatment.

c **False**

The hypersomnolence is probably indicative of CO_2 retention when uncontrolled O_2 therapy would be contraindicated (at least until full assessment)

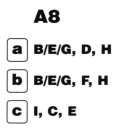

d **False**

Although possible, an unlikely sole cause in view of the breathlessness unless associated with profound obesity. It may however complicate COPD when the tendency to obstructive sleep apnoea (OSA) will further increase nocturnal desaturation and secondary polycythaemia. It is this rather than cyanosis that is probably alarming his wife

A8

a B/E/G, D, H

b B/E/G, F, H

c I, C, E

A9

a **False**

A grade II response is consistent with vaccination with BCG or post infection and not typical of active disease

b **True**

Although the danger of this has been exaggerated re-expansion pulmonary oedema does seem to occur more frequently when the lung re-expands rapidly after having been deflated for some time. This rarely occurs in malignancy and larger volumes can be safely drained although cough and mediastinal discomfort is fairly common. It probably is sensible to limit drainage to 1-2 litres over 2-3 hours and then leave on free drainage

c **True**

Depending on cytologist, pleural fluid is positive 30-60%, whilst Abrahamís biopsy is less than 10% positive (and frequently contains little pleura!)

d **True**

90% undiagnosed pleural effusions will be diagnosed following thoracoscopy which is infrequently requested! A true diagnosis of non-specific pleurisy is more easily accepted than a similar report resulting from a blind biopsy

A10

a **False**

The history is not of a serious (life threatening) community acquired pneumonia – the only indication for combined therapy although this is commonly prescribed in patients with exacerbation of COPD!

b **False**

A negative result may reflect cell mediated immune suppression resulting from renal failure although a strongly positive result would be useful

c **True**

Hospital-acquired or opportunist infection is possible in this patient and lung lavage provides more specific microbiological results than sputum

d **False**

Renal failure of this degree requires omission of ethambutol and dose reduction of other drugs

A11

a **True**

This combination does not provide sufficient anaerobic cover and inadequate for staph lung infection

b **False**

An aspiration pneumonia with cavitation is more likely with this history.

c **False**

Isolation of staph from the mouth is common following broad spectrum antibiotics and this commonly contaminates sputum. It may be significant however

d **False**

No risk factors identified in history

A12

a **True**

Conventional advice is to abandon aspiration if air still being aspirated after two litres have been removed

b **True (probably)**

The chances of a recurrence progressively increases by 15% after first occurrence, 50% following the second and more than 70% after the third. A chemical pleurodesis (with tetracycline) is an alternative but less satisfactory method to pleural stripping or talc insuflation. With increasing air travel and as pleurodesis is now a minor procedure it is being recommended at an earlier stage than previously.

c **False**

Underlying lung disease such as bullous emphysema is likely, ie this is not a spontaneous uncomplicated case

d **False**

Conventional treatment would be to employ suction and delay surgery by 10-14 days. In some centres, particularly mainland Europe, assessment by thoracoscope would lead to early surgical intervention if lung 'blebs' are seen

e **False**

This will occur if the tube has migrated out of the pleural cavity or is blocked with fibrin. If the lung is re-expanded and remains so overnight, the tube may be removed

A13

a Both CXR and ECG will be performed but may be unhelpful. CXR can show relative paucity of blood vessels or a wedge-shaped infarct which radiography are characteristic. ECG may show acute right heart strain which suggests haemodynamically significant embolism

Venous ultrasonography of the leg is indicated – high sensitivity and specificity for proximal clot – many radiology departments now offer this as a 'screening service'

ABGs are conventionally requested but the degree of hypoxaemia is poorly related to size or risk from embolism. Contrary to common belief, 'normal' ABGs do not exclude pulmonary embolism, especially recurrent minor emboli. V/Q scanning not required urgently and probably unnecessary when clinical suspicion is high as in this case. Treatment or further investigation should not be delayed while awaiting V/Q scan

Measurement of D dimers is very helpful and will exclude thrombo-embolism when normal but an elevated value in this case would be useful. Commercial kits have made this test more readily available

Echocardiography should be performed in the A&E department if there is evidence of low cardiac output or symptoms to suggest major embolism. In this case it might be requested to evalute the degree of pulmonary hypertension ie clinical importance of further thrombo-embolism

b Previous history would include need for procoagulant screening such as protein C and S deficiency, Leiden V abnormality or lupus coagulant

Pregnancy or use of oral contraceptive. So-called third generation oestrogen oral contraceptives have an increased risk of thrombo-embolism compared with second generation OCs. This risk is multiplied 30 fold if there is a procoagulant condition

A history of GI haemorrhage, previous SAH or other relative contraindication to anticoagulation or thrombolysis

A14

a **False**

The decision to intubate is primarily based upon clinical features and progress (or lack of progress) with initial treatment not on a predetermined abnormality in ABG. Nevertheless a severe respiratory acidosis eg pH < 7.25, pCO_2 > 10.0kPa will require intubation unless secondary to complicating pneumothorax or other immediately remedial cause

b **False**

Aminophylline is being abandoned in favour of either IV beta-agonists or simply increased frequency of nebuliser therapy. Trials have indicated no additional benefit with aminophylline but significant morbidity, particularly status epilepticus, especially when oral therapy may have unknowingly been taken prior to hospital attendance

c **False**

Although NIV can be successfully employed in asthma this patient has a prolonged history suggestive of airway inflammation and oedema which will take some days to settle rather than acute bronchospasm, the so called 'clear blue sky' asthma. The latter may present with repeated near fatal attacks that improve rapidly and can be managed with NIV, if clinicians are experienced. A second reason is that he is agitated – NIV requires patient co-operative which is unlikely in the present case

d **False**

With evidence of impending ventilatory failure (elevated pCO_2) it would be regarded as unacceptable to use a sedative and could not be defended if the patient suffered a respiratory arrest. Asthmatics should only be sedated when intubated and on controlled mechanical ventilation

e **True**

There are numerous case reports, but no controlled studies, of the value of IV magnesium which acts as bronchodilator by relaxing smooth muscle. 10-20 mmols IV over 30 mins is worth trying in extremis.

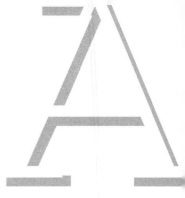

GROUP 12: ITU

A1

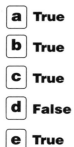

a True

b False

c True

d True

e False

A2

a True

b True

c True

d False

e True

A3

a True

b False

c True

d False

e True

A4

a True

b True

c False

d True

e True

A5

The history is often helpful, eg pneumonia, UTI, bleeding, previous peptic ulcer disease, chest pain, previous ischaemic episode. Pre-operative assessment is vital in patients undergoing non-cardiac surgery to prevent cardiogenic complications leading to shock. Clinical risk factors include a high-risk surgical procedure, a history of ischaemic or cerebral vascular disease, a history of Type I diabetes, and a pre-operative serum creatinine over 177 μmoles/l.

In hypovolaemic shock the BP is often maintained initially but hypotension invariably occurs. In cardiogenic shock the venous pressure is raised and there may be pulsus alternans and a gallop rhythm; these are usually signs of pulmonary oedema . In septicaemic shock there is pyrexia often with rigors, vasodilatation, warm peripheries and a bounding pulse.

A6

The first feature is often an unexplained tachypnoea followed by increasing hypoxaemia, dyspnoea and laboured breathing. Fine crackles are heard throughout both lung fields. The CXR shows bilateral diffuse alveolar shadowing sometimes with air bronchogram. There is no cardiac enlargement.

The management consists of the treatment of the underlying cause. The outcome in ARDS is directly related to this and not the initial severity of the lung lesion. Respiratory support, using synchronised, intermittent, mandatory ventilation (SIMV) or pressure limited ventilation are better than conventional mehtods of ventilation, particularly with high levels of PEEP. Prognosis is very dependent on the aetiology. When associated with septic shock, mortality rates are as high as 90%, many dying from multiple organ dysfunctional syndrome (MODS).

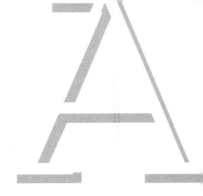

GROUP 13: Poisoning

A1

a | True
b | False
c | True
d | True
e | False

A2

a | False
b | True
c | True
d | False
e | True

A3

a | False
b | True
c | True
d | True
e | False

A4

a | The blood gases show a respiratory alkalosis due to hyperventilation; a direct effect of aspirin on the ventilatory centre. Subsequent compensatory mechanisms include renal extraction of bicarbonate and potassium which result in a metabolic acidosis and a rise in [H+] concentration.

b Aspirin. This is, by far, the commonest cause of this clinical picture due to poisoning.

c Questions to ask include: Was there a clear precipitant cause? Was the act premeditated or impulsive? Did the patient leave a suicide note? Had the patient taken pains not to be discovered? What are the patient's feelings about the suicide attempt now?

A5

General management principles of an overdose

Cardiac monitoring

Give activated charcoal

IV fluid should consist of normal saline. Glucose may worsen the hypokalaemia

Specific therapy with digoxin antibody fragments are used in the following:

serum potassium > 6mmoles/l;

digoxin level > 10 nmoles/l, six hours after drug ingestion;

life-threatening dysrhythmias, eg ventricular tachycardia;

cardiac decompensation

A6

True

A7

Paracetamol

Aspirin

Benzodiazepines

A8

Ibuprofen

Iron

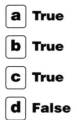

A9

<1%

A10

Prompt airways management

Satisfactory oxygenation as required

Maintenance of stable CVS

Careful and close nursing and medical monitoring

Poison centre advice 24 hours a day

Psychiatric support if required

A11

a **True**

b Alcohol

A12

a **True**

b **True**

c **True**

d **False**

A13

< 4 hours

A14

Use active charcoal – to reduce absorption

Enhance elimination – check with Poison's Unit

A15

False

A16

Aspirin

Theophylline

Anti-convulsants

A17

Erythromycin and other macrolides - because of risk of increasing QT time

A18

Aspirin

Dapsone

Mercury

Theophyllines

A19

Naloxone is the antidote for opiates and is indicated in overdose when the patient is drowsy

Desferrioximine is the antidote for Fe salts and is indicated in all confirmed cases of Fe overdose

Flumazenil is the antidote for benzodiazepine and is indicated in overdose with drowsiness

A20

Yes – the patient is at risk of death

Ecstacy usage is common but the incidence of overdose is low

A21

a BP, Pulse, PR, O_2, Temp and emergency bedside testing of capillary glucose

b FBC

Biochemistry (U&Es, creatinine, LFTs, glucose & cardiac enzymes)

Drug screen

Urinalysis for myoglobin

Clotting screen

c Paracetamol

Aspirin

Alcohol

Benzodiazepines

Opiates

Tricyclic anti-depressants

d Half hourly neuro-observations

Nurse in left lateral position

Hourly BP/pulse/temp/respiratory rate/sat O_2/urine output

Ensure on correct pressure relief bedding

Transfer to a HDU area

e She should remain on ECG monitoring continuously until recovered

A22

a The first patient ingested within four hours is likely to have little or no symptoms and may eventually ask to go home on the same day

The second patient may well develop symptoms, eg nausea, vomiting, anorexia, RU abdominal pain, abdominal tenderness on exam. The patient may well be developing liver failure

b The patient less than four hours after OD should have the paracetamol level checked in two hours time. Thereafter, N-acetylcysteine (NAC) may be commenced based on the normogram. (See BNF)

The second patient should have a paracetamol level checked and NAC is often given but its effectiveness is questionable

| c | Yes, because high-risk patients may benefit from NAC infusion beyond 24 hours

after ingestion

| d | Discuss with liver unit

| e | U&E/Creatinine raised due to hepato-renal syndrome

INR (prothrombin time) because most sensitive marker of ongoing liver dysfunction

LFTs because Bilirubin, AST and ALT will rise initially and then fall either because the patient has progressed to fuliminant hepatic failure (FHF) or they have recovered

FBC is not indicated unless there is bleeding and paracetamol level is of no value

A23

Transfer to liver unit for possible transplantation

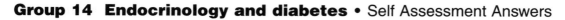

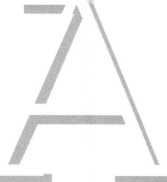

GROUP 14: Endocrinology and diabetes

A1

a **False**

Uptake is increased

b **True**

Uptake is reduced

c **False**

Antithyroid drugs block iodine incorporation, but not uptake

d **True**

The virus in de Quervains thyroiditis disrupts the uptake mechanism of thyroid cells, and turns the cells into virus replicators rather than thyroxine synthesisers.

e **True**

Radioiodine uptake is always reduced in viral thyroiditis. The patient becomes thyrotoxic because all the stored thyroxine in the thyroid gland is released acutely as the thyroid is damaged. Once this is metabolised, the patient becomes hypothyroid as no thyroxine is being synthesised. Resolution occurs (like in any viral disease) two to four months later

f **True**

Amiodarone has got large amounts of iodine, and therefore radioiodine uptake is reduced

g **True**

Amiodarone has a half life of over a month, so there is no significant uptake for several months after amiodarone is discontinued

A2

a Thyroid storm. Although the cause of the pyrexia and the tachycardia may be due to the pneumonia and the heart failure, this patient has thyroid storm by definition.

b Beta blockers should be added in addition to the usual treatment for pneumonia and heart failure (antibiotics and diuretics). Rate control with beta blockers (to a rate of 150 but no lower) is essential

c Intensive care. Mortality is 50% if the thyrotoxicosis is not treated, and very careful fluid monitoring is essential. This will usually require central venous catheterisation, because of the risk of precipitating pulmonary oedema

d Cool the patient and replace fluids

Give propranolol 40mg, eight hourly

Propyl-thiouracil 250mg, four hourly followed after at least one hour by potassium iodide 60mg eight hourly, if the storm is not controlled by previous measures

A3

Lie patient down

Intravenous normal saline, until no postural drop

Intramuscular hydrocortisone 100mg, then orally

Oral fludrocortisone 100mcg

Intravenous or oral glucose if hypoglycaemic

A4

Primary hyperparathyroidism

A5

This patient should have her blood pressure measured regularly, to look for resultant carpal spasm. If this does occur, the patient has a positive Trousseau's sign, and should have calcium replacement. If the patient has had long standing hyperparathyroidism previously, she may have 'hungry bones' which will continue to remove calcium from the plasma now that the PTH excess has been removed, so calcium replacement may need to be prolonged. If the hypocalcaemia does not respond, the patient may need support with alfacalcidol. Patients are managed with a lowish calcium (2.20-2.30mmol/l) in the hope that this will stimulate PTH synthesis from the remaining parathyroid glands

A6

a In a patient who is found to have four gland hyperplasia, one must consider an inherited cause of hyperparathyroidism, such as multiple endocrine neoplasia

b This patient will need lifelong alfacalcidol, because she has no remaining parathyroid tissue. One of the actions of PTH is to activate renal one-alpha hydroxylase, and this clearly cannot occur

c Patients should be run with a low normal calium level (2.20-2.30mmol/l), in order to minimise the risk of renal stones, which occur more commonly in patients requiring alfacalcidol. Unlike PTH (which increases calcium and reduces phosphate), alfacalcidol increases both calcium and phosphate, thus increasing the risk of renal stones

A7

a **False**

Papillary thyroid carcinoma has no relationship with phaeochromocytomas

b **True**

Medullary thyroid carcinoma may be part of multiple endocrine neoplasia type 2 which is an autosomally dominantly inherited condition

c **False**

Papillary thyroid carcinoma has no relationship with phaeochromocytomas

d **True**

Medullary thyroid carcinoma may be part of multiple endocrine neoplasia type 2 which is an autosomally dominantly inherited condition

e **True**

f **True**

g **False**

A8

a **True**

The pituitary secretes large amounts of ACTH in response to adrenal failure. ACTH is synthesised as POMC (pro-opio melanocortin) which is cleaved to several peptides, including endorphins and enkephalins

b **True**

Cushing's disease is the commonest cause of endogenous Cushing's syndrome, and is caused by a pituitary tumour that secretes ACTH

c **False**

Postural hypotension does not occur in patients with pituitary infarction, because aldosterone rather than cortisol is primarily in control of postural blood pressure. Aldosterone is controlled by the renin-angiotensin system rather than the pituitary. Addison's disease results in loss of both cortisol and aldosterone

d **False**

The male pituitary does not become ischaemic, as it has an excellent blood supply. Patients who have pituitary infarction will not survive, as this will be associated with cerebral ischaemia

e **False**

At the end of pregnancy, the pituitary is critically ischaemic, even with a normal blood pressure. This is because the pituitary gland enlarges significantly during pregnancy, but its blood supply cannot, as it comes through the hypothalamus. Only a small fall (not hypovolaemic shock) is required to cause pituitary infarction

A9

Psychogenic polydipsia. Lithium is known to cause nephrogenic diabetes insipidus (with dilute urine), but this would clearly result in a high plasma sodium (and a high but ineffective ADH level in the blood if it is measured). This patient has neither DI (which would result in a high rather than a low plasma sodium) nor SIADH (which would result in a high urine specific gravity)

A10

a **True**

This is DKA

b **True**

This is hyperosmaolar non-ketotic coma (HONKC).

c **True**

d **False**

Metformin is an insulin sensitiser and never causes hypoglycaemia. It is well known to cause lactic acidosis either in overdose, or in patients who are in renal failure, where metformin can accumulate

e **False**

Patients inapproriately being advised to stop their insulin is one of the commonest causes of DKA

f **True**

They are NOT insulin dependent.

g **True**

After a dose of glucagon, hepatic glycogen must be replenished by giving the patient a carbohydate rich meal

h **True**

As pregnancy progresses, patients become more and more insulin resistant

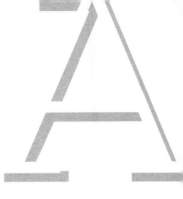

GROUP 15: Neurology

A1

a Meningococcal meningitis is, by far, the most likely diagnosis

b Immediate benzylpenicillin 2.4g every four-to-six hours by slow IV injection or by infusion. If she had been seen by a doctor prior to coming to A&E she should have been given IM or IV benzylpenicillin 1.2g immediately. If she was allergic to penicillin she should have been given cefotaxime

c A blood culture will show the meningococcus but do not delay in giving the antibiotics. A lumbar puncture is not necessary in a patient with meningitis and a purpuric rash

d Give rifampicin 600mg twice daily for two days

Household and other close contacts should also be given the drug

You should notify the case

Other students should be recommended to be immunised by plain polysaccharide A&C vaccine

A2

a True

b False

c False

d True

e True

An isolated VI nerve palsy occurs in diabetes due to an infarction. It is a common sequel of head trauma. In raised intracranial pressure the VI nerve is compressed against the petrous temporal bone.

A3

a The mild spastic quadriparesis suggests a cervical cord lesion, probably due to cervical spondylosis. The buttock pain on walking with good peripheral pulses suggests spinal stenosis. The absent ankle jerks localises this to the L5/S1 level

b An MRI of the neck and lower spine should be performed. If necessary, electrophysiological studies could confirm the functional significance of the lesions seen

c Most cases of cervical spondylosis can be managed conservatively with analgesics and a cervical collar. Surgical decompression is advised if there is no progression of the symptoms and signs. Spinal stenosis in the lumbar area frequently does well with surgery

A4

Cataract. WHO estimates that 32 million operations would have to be done yearly by 2020 to reduce the problem to zero

Trachoma due to Chlamydia trachomatis. Treatment involves early surgery because trichiasis (internal eyelashes scratching the cornea) is the main cause of blindness. Antibiotics, facial cleanliness and control of flies are also an important part of the strategy

Onchocerciasis. This filarial disease can be treated with ivermectin. This does not kill the adult worms, which can live for many years. One single dose per year keeps the larvae down to minimal numbers and prevents blindness

A5

a Proximal myopathy

Sensory peripheral neuropathy

b The proximal myopathy (which is often easily missed) in the setting of abnormal liver biochemistry is strongly suggestive of alcohol abuse. The absent ankle jerks and sensory abnormalities and the raised MCV also suggest alcohol abuse which this lady eventually admitted

A6

A central feature of the regulations is that it is illegal to drive a motor vehicle in the UK if any form of seizure has taken place in the previous year. It is an essential requirement of you, as a doctor, to inform these patients of the regulations. The patient should write to the licensing authorities. These regulations apply whether the patient is on or off treatment. Regulations for vocational and truck drivers are stricter and they must meet all of the following three criteria

They must have been free of epileptic attacks for the last ten years

They must not have taken anti-convulsants during the ten year period

They do not have a continuing liability to epileptic seizures

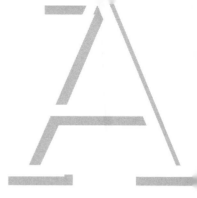

GROUP 16: Psychiatry

A1

a **False**

Most deliberate self harm is not associated with a major psychiatric disorder. Many occur after a life event with up to half associated with relationship difficulties

b **False**

Patients who present with DSH have a greatly increased risk of suicide during the following year compared with the general population

c **True**

Around one-fifth of DSH presentations are motivated by serious suicidal intentions. Other motivations include temporary escape from overwhelming stress or to effect a change in personal circumstances

d **False**

In up to 50% of cases deliberate self harm is associated with recent alcohol consumption

e **False**

The commonest presentation is self poisoning

A2

a **True**

Many completed suicides are associated with a psychiatric illness, most often major depression

b **True**

Psychotic symptoms (eg delusions, hallucination) suggest more severe psychotic disturbance and increased suicide risk

c **False**

Higher risk groups include the elderly and young males

d **True**

Chronic painful illness can also be associated with other risk factors, eg spousal isolation, unemployment, older age

e **False**

Marital status is considered to be of protective value with respect to suicide

A3

a Persecutory delusions are associated with a number of psychiatric disorders. In a patient with advanced physical disease the most likely diagnoses are delirium and psychotic depression, although a previous major psychiatric diagnosis, eg schizophrenia, would also be relevant.

b Disorientation in time and place with clouding of consciousness are characteristic of delirium though not always consistent. Other features include visual illusions and hallucinations (which are uncommon in other psychotic illnesses), persecutory delusions and fear. Behaviour is unpredictable and may change through the day

c In the history of relevance are onset and duration of disturbed behaviour and persecutory ideas, previous psychiatric history, current medication and history of alcohol misuse. Important investigations include:

Full blood screen, U&E, Ca, blood sugar, liver and cardiac enzymes

ECG (silent infarct)

CT Brain scan

EEG – may show excess slow waves and be helpful when clinical presentation unclear

Infection screen (MSU, CXR, blood and sputum culture)

d Management of delirium includes:

Nursing: safe, low stimulation environment

Maintain hydration, nutrition

Treat underlying cause

Keep drugs to a minimum

Symptomatic treatment of psychotic symptoms (delusions, hallucinations) and any associated disturbed behaviour with antipsychotic drugs starting at low dose and avoiding strong anticholinergic medications, eg haloperidol 1.5-5mg up to three times daily. If extrapyramidal side-effects occur, newer antipsychotics may be used

A4

Features include

Psychomotor retardation or agitation

Low mood

Intedonia (loss of interest or pleasure)

Reduced energy and motivation

Suicidal thoughts which should always be explored

Depressive thinking (pessimism, guilt, worthlessness, self reproach, hopelessness – often associated with suicidal thoughts)

Biological symptoms (early wakening, diurnal mood variation, reduced appetite and weight)

In the most severe cases mood congruent delusions and perceptual abnormalities (eg auditory hallucinations) may be present (psychotic depression)

An urgent psychiatric assessment is indicated if patient is at risk, eg suicidal, not eating or drinking, psychotic symptoms present (treatment may be required under the Mental Health Act)

A5

a False

Opiate withdrawal is not usually associated with convulsions unless complicated by withdrawal from other substances such as alcohol or tranquillisers (benzodiazepines, barbiturates)

b False

Naloxone reverses the effects of opiate intoxication and can rapidly bring on the acute withdrawal syndrome

c False

Methadone has a longer half life than heroin (allowing once daily dosing). The withdrawal syndrome can take longer to become evident and be more prolonged though possibly less intense

d False

The opiate withdrawal syndrome is characterised by physical symptoms and some objectively evident signs (eg pupilary dilation, rhinorrhoea, lacrimation, sweating, piloerection)

e False

Uncomplicated opiate withdrawal is subjectively unpleasant and distressing but rarely life threatening

A6

a

The symptoms suggest extrapyramidal side-effects of the antipsychotic medication which are common with older 'typical' antipsychotic agents and less often seen with the newer so-called 'atypical' antipsychotics. Acute extrapyramidal symptoms (EPS) include 'pseudoparkinsonism' as evident in this case, acute dystonia (involuntary muscular contractions involving neck, limbs, trunk or face) and oculogyric crises characterised by abnormal eye movements

b

Following a full physical examination to exclude any other organic problem requiring further exploration, acute extrapyramidamal symptoms can be reversed by administering an anticholinergic drug such as procyclidine (5-10mg). The intramuscular or intravenous route can achieve faster relief of the symptoms such as acute dystonia. In the longer term consider regular oral anticholinergic drug (eg procyclidine 5mg bd), reduction in antipsychotic dose or changing to an atypical antipsychotic

c An uncommon but serious idiosyncratic reaction to antipsychotic medication (occurring in around 0.5% of newly treated patients with a 15% mortality) is the neuroleptic malignant syndrome (NMS) the signs of which include pyrexia, severe muscle rigidity, autonomic instability and clouded consciousness. It is more frequently associated with high potency antipsychotics such as haloperidol. Further clues to the diagnosis are a very high creatine phosphokinase, raised white cell count and ESR

d Exclude other possible causes of delirium. Mortality in NMS is often due to cardiac arrest (due to autonomic dysfunction) or renal failure. Urgent inpatient medical attention is required, if necessary intensive care. All antipsychotic medication must be stopped, hydration, electrolyte status, renal and cardiac function monitored closely and cardiorespiratory support made available. Anticholinergic medication is not indicated. Other supportive measures can include administering dantrolene (muscle relaxant) and the dopamine agonist bromocriptine may be considered to reverse the effects of central dopaminergic blockade caused by the antipsychotic drug

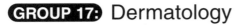

GROUP 17: Dermatology

A1

Points to be covered: It is very rare; it is very very severe (30% to 50% mortality); it normally needs ITU care; the blisters lead to denuding of most or all skin; there is a loss of internal epithelium; it is commonly caused by drugs or is idiopathic in origin

A2

Points to be covered: it is a complication of atopic eczema, there is widespread HSV skin infection; the clinical picture is early vesicles, leading to punched out crusted erosions on any body site, but face and around the eye is common; the patient is often unwell with pyrexia, unlike in bacterial infected eczema; it is very rarely lethal if not treated; it is normally one-off but can be recurrent; prescribe oral aciclovir; if unwell or pyrexial, IV aciclovir is indicated; also prescribe for secondary bacterial infection (flucloxacillin with or without penicillin V), and prescribe emollients and topical steroids

A3

Erythema multiforme

TEN

Pemphigus

Pemphigoid

Lichen planus

Reiter syndrome

Behcet's syndrome/disease

HIV sero-conversion illness

SLE

A4

Interdigital spaces (tinea pedis)

Soles of feet (fissured hyperkeratotic eczema)

Surprisingly leg ulcer is a rare cause of cellulitis. Most develop de novo with no obvious predisposing cause but tinea pedis skin maceration is often present. On examination, the patient is pyrexial and feels very unwell. The skin may blister. Malaise++ is very common in cellulitis

A5

DVT

Cellulitis

Ruptured Baker's cyst

Lipodermatosclerosis (LDS)

Lipodermatosclerosis is common in people with chronic venous insufficiency. It may not be associated with venous leg ulcers. LDS can present as a firm, woody, hot, red brown swelling. It tends to present at the ankle. Unlike cellulitis it stays localised and is not associated with malaise and pyrexia. Treatment is with compression not antibiotics

A6

Strep titres (ASOT)

FBC

ESR

Blood sugar

Skin/throat swabs and blood cultures rarely of any use

A7

Necrotising fasciitis. This is rare but much commoner in diabetes. It can occur de novo or post surgery. It is an emergency as it will not respond to antibiotics. Urgent surgical exploration and extensive debridement is needed. Amputation can be life-saving. Treatment of cellulitis usually needs three-to-four days IV antibiotics and ten days oral antibiotics or recurrence rate is high

A8

a You specifically want to ask a detailed drug history, history of breathing problems, TB contact, bowel symptoms. Prior history of sore throat, previous BCG vaccination, living abroad

b One could argue in the absence of any history suggesting an underlying cause extensive investigations are unnecessary. Many cases are idiopathic or due to sarcoidosis and resolve spontaneously. The basic investigations are: Strep titres (ASOT); throat swab; CXR; 1/10,000 Mantoux test. If there is a rash elsewhere or there is a neuropathy a dermatology referral is indicated. Consider leprosy (a common cause world wide), if the patient is from an endemic area

c By elevation/bed rest/tubigrip and NSAIDS. If rash persists or ulcerates refer to dermatology for dapsone, prednisolone or colchicine

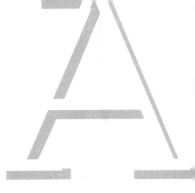

A9

a Drug ingestion, including recreational, homeopathic and vitamins

Dietary history, especially recent seafood, peanuts, strawberries, 'new food'

Past history skin disease

Photosensitivity

Recent infection, URTI, D&V etc

Recent travel abroad

b Urticaria, most likely idiopathic, and angioedema. Rare underlying causes include food, drugs, viral/parasitic infection, subacute LE

c Explain condition is idiopathic, what this means and why, therefore, tests are not needed. Most cases last weeks, occasionally months to years. Treat with non-sedating anti-histamine

d No. Hereditary angio-oedema (HAE) causes angioedema but not urticaria. However, a morbilliform maculopapuler rash may preceed an attack of angioderma

A10

a Erythema multiforme major. Ask dermatology to see him.

b Pemphigoid (but he's a bit young and oral lesions are not common)

Pemphigus (usually presents with hyperkeratotic erosions and little in the way of blisters as they rupture easily)

Bullous lichen planus. Normally very itchy lesions are purplish with white streaking scale on surface

c Bullous impetigo (often very crusted)

Pompholyx eczema (hands and feet very common sites), very very itchy

Staphylococcal scalded skin syndrome (widespread background, erythema, skin often comes off in sheets)

Other causes of blisters include: HSV and VZV (more localised, blisters rupture early and leave painful crusted erosions); insect bites (papular urticaria - localised and clustered); burns; cellulitis; TEN

d Farmer is a sheep farmer. Orf disease on his hand, leading to secondary erythema multiforme

e Idiopathic >50% (see list in Kumar & Clark)

Causes include:

Herpes simplex virus (the most common identifiable cause)

Other viral infections (eg EBV, Orf disease)

Drugs (eg sulphonamide, barbiturates)

Mycoplasma infection

Connective tissue disease (eg SLE, classical polyarteritis nodosa)

HIV infection

Wegener's granulomatosus

Carcinoma, lymphoma

f If not eating and drinking - admit. Give IV fluids and analgesia. Start oral steroids early but this is controversial, aseptic mouth washes, oral hygiene. Resolves in two to four weeks.

Notes on nomenclature

EM minor - lesions, target lesions, often palms, soles, no mucosal involvement

EM major - mucosal involvement

Stevens Johnson Syndrome – mild form TEN, mucosal and eye involvement, few blisters on skin, no target lesion

TEN – severe and internal mucosal involvement (lung, gut, bladder), blisters, shedding off huge areas of skin

A11

a Check rectal temperature – likely hypothermic

Space blanket to warm up

Blood cultures

U&Es, urgent dermatology referral

Rehydrate

Check cardiac stability

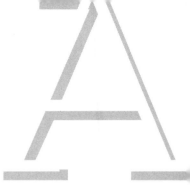

b Erythrodermic pustular psoriasis (common in alcoholics)

Anti-convulsant hypersensitivity syndrome (ACHS)

c ACHS usually occurs within two-to-three weeks of starting anti-convulsants

There is often eosinophilia

Swinging very high temperature

Lymphadenopathy

Deranged LFTS

Skin biopsy should also help

d see BLM

e Valproate, not phenytoin or lamotrigine, which cross react as they have a similar chemical structure

Warning

Erythroderma involving 90% or more of the skin is an emergency and requires resuscitation and hospital admission with urgent dermatology referral

A12

a Scabies

Eczema (atopic) as known atopic but distribution usually flexural

Dermatitis herpetiformis (distribution usually buttocks and elbows – blisters only seen in early disease)

b Anyone living with him affected/unaffected?

Were they treated at same time as him even if unaffected?

Partner (regular or otherwise) affected?

How did he use the prescription?

c Any person living with him must be treated even if unaffected as they may be carriers. Scabies is transmitted by close contact (living with or sexual)

Occasionally resistance is seen to malathion. Consider alternative, eg permethrin

Repeated scabies prescription leads to irritant dermatitis. Patients should be warned itch can go on for one month after successful treatment of scabies. Therefore give some crotamiton rather than further scabies prescription

All of the skin below the neck must be treated, including genitals, under nails and soles of feet